DISABILITY
TOWARDS INCLUSIVE INDIA

DISABILITY
TOWARDS INCLUSIVE INDIA

Edited by

Dr. Ruchi Ramesh
Dr. Sudhir Kumar Singh

In Association with
SOCIETY FOR SOCIAL EMPOWERMENT, NEW DELHI

PENTAGON PRESS

Disability: Towards Inclusive India
Dr. Ruchi Ramesh, Dr. Sudhir Kumar Singh (*Eds.*)

ISBN 978-81-8274-566-7

First Published in 2011

Published by

PENTAGON PRESS
206, Peacock Lane, Shahpur Jat
New Delhi-110049
Phones: 011-64706243, 26491568
Telefax: 011-26490600
email: rajan@pentagonpress.in
website: www.pentagonpress.in

Printed at Himal Impressions, New Delhi.

Contents

Preface

The concept of human rights is gaining momentum day by day at the global level. International community has witnessed the unprecedented growth of this movement after the end of the cold war. India has not been aloof from this international process of the protection and promotion of the cardinal values of human rights. At the national level in last few decades we have lifted 300 million people from the poverty line but still 300 million people are languishing under poverty line. It is one of the most important challenges for the Indian democracy. It has been projected from various quarters that India would be a strong country within next few decades. If we have to ensure sustainable development, we have to bring all marginalized sectors into mainstream. The most unfortunate and hapless people are that of disabled community within marginalized groups. They are facing twin problem of social apathy as well as state negligence. They have remained an important victim of our negligence.

Disability has emerged as an important component of the development process across the globe in recent period. The post cold war system has given a new twist to the notion of human rights and the plight of the PWD has been highlighted accordingly. Disable community is compelled to face the twin problem of social discrimination as well as governmental apathy. There are varieties of disability, some are by born and many surface after the birth due to gamut of reasons. In 2007 the United Nations has passed a new Convention for the protection and promotion of the rights of the disabled community. India is also one of the signatories of this convention therefore India is also compelled to implement all welfare measures included in UN Convention.

Despite numerous policies and statements regarding disability and poverty reduction, it is still estimated that globally 50,000 people, including 10,000 disabled people, die every day as a result of chronic poverty. This is not an abstract theory, but a disastrous crisis. Majority among this ratio of hapless people belong to the developing countries. Despite all round progress India still remains developing country and health care still remains one of the major concerns for India. Majority of Indians remain in the rural sector, which has neither sufficient health amenities nor means of speedy travel to the cities where medicinal facilities are available.

India still has around 30 per cent poor people, who live below the poverty line. Our developmental process has not been able to accommodate this component of interlink age between disability and poverty. The relationship between disability and poverty is often described as a vicious circle. Here, it is argued that in fact, both disability and poverty are often manifestations of the same process. If the commonalities are recognized then the need to build horizontal alliances becomes more apparent.

According to the NSSO 2002 survey, around only 26 per cent disables are employed. Out of the total disable population 50 per cent or little more are in employable age (20-60 years). It has also been revealed by the survey that around 60 per cent of the disabled can take care of themselves without aids and appliances and another about 17 per cent can carry on daily activities of life with aids and appliances. It means that around 77 per cent disable population is able for executing works for economic emancipation. This is a good sign that due to general health improvement and various measures especially through health interventions taken by the Government, prevalence and incidence of disability specially visual disability, hearing and speech disabilities have come down when findings of 47th and 58th Round of NSSO surveys are compared.

The 1986 UN Declaration of the Right of the Development has proclaimed that right to development is also an integral part of the fundamental human rights. The proper right to development could not be realized by the disable community without employment opportunities. This is extremely tough challenge before us, which at any cost have to be fulfilled for the larger interest of these helpless brothers and sisters of our society.

The Government of India is a signatory to international agreements and has several poverty alleviation initiatives aimed specifically to the disabled community. These schemes however have only reinforced the cycle of dependence of the disabled. They view disability in isolation and fail to see the linkage with other forms of marginalization. For instance NSSO data 1991 indicates that about 40 per cent of the disabled belong to the SC/ST community. Economic marginalization and disability are also inter-related.

The gender component is also very pertinent here. Given the horizontal linkage of disability with other forms of marginalization it is imperative that a disability perspective is incorporated in the governmental policies, especially in the 11th Five Year Plan in consonance with the decision to incorporate a gender dimension.

This book is intended to emphasize the interlinkage between poverty, disability and human rights. The scholars of diverse backgrounds have contributed their articles in this proceeding targeting some of most thorny issues confronted by the disable community today. Employment has emerged as an important instrument to bring the disable community into the mainstreaming process of the development. For disable community it is more relevant because the disable community requires more economic protection to cope with its extra requirements. This community is deprived at the front of human rights. A sustainable India could not emerge till we do not provide due space for the genuine grievances of the disable community.

Dr. Ruchi Ramesh
Dr. Sudhir Kumar Singh

About the Contributors

Col (retd.) Anil Bhat was in Indian military and currently reputed columnist on strategic issues based in New Delhi.

Dr. Alok Kumar Gupta is Associate Professor, National Law University, Ranchi.

Dr. Amit Rahul is working with a think tank based in New Delhi.

Dr. Asha J.V. is Assistant Professor, University of Kerela.

Dr. Bhupinder Zutshi is Associate Professor, CSRD, Jawaharlal Nehru University, New Delhi.

Sri. C. Ravi Sankar is Assistant Professor, Andhra University, Vishakhaptnam.

Ms. Geetanjali Sharma is a Research Scholar at National Law University, Jodhpur.

Dr. Jayadeba Sahoo is Associate Professor, Rajiv Gandhi University, Itanagar, Arunachal Pradesh.

Mr. Pankaj Sreshakar is Deputy Secretary, Central Information Commission, Government of India, New Delhi.

Dr. Ruchi Ramesh is Associate Professor, Department of Sociology, R.K.M.V. Shimla, Himachal Pradesh.

Dr. Rakesh Raman Jha is disable right activist based in New Delhi.

Mrs Rashmi Sharma is teaching in CCS University, Merrut.

Ms. Rashmi Sinha is working with a think tank based in New Delhi.

Dr. S. Prabhakar is Deputy Director, Lok-Sabha, New Delhi.

Dr. P. Saibabu is Associate Professor, Andhra University, Vishkhapatnam.

Dr. Sudhir Kumar Singh is Assistant Professor, Department of Political Science, Dyal Singh College, University of Delhi, New Delhi.

Dr. Vandana Bhardawaj is teaching in CCS University, Merrut.

Dr. Vivek Saini is an independent scholar based in New Delhi.

Introduction

Disability remains at the periphery within the process of development across the globe. There is no difference of developed or developing countries even in this direction. However within the developed countries the system of social security under the broader framework of welfare state concept as one of the important instruments of democracy works and it has provided them economic security at extent. But even in these societies disable people are subject to social apathy and that has not been achieved till the society at large will not be able to understand that disable people are also part and parcel of the society and their dignity must be protected and respected at par with able people. The concept of human security, human rights, justice, equality, liberty are considered as the foundation of any vibrant democratic system but unfortunately within democratic societies even the disable people's rights have not been adequately respected due to variety of reasons. In developing countries the disable community confronted with the twin problem of social and economic deprivation and thus remained far away from the mainstreaming process of the development. They have not been considered equal by practical sense by the state and by the society but they have of course paid lip services for their all round development. Globally the number of disable people constitutes 1/10 of the overall population and it has been an established fact that without their incorporation into the mainstreaming process of development, no society could achieve the notion of sustainable development. The dynamics of the situation of the disable people is different in India because government of India is not conceding its actual number and putting its number between 2-3 per cent of the overall population. While government of India estimates of prevalence of disability is low, alternative estimates using better methods and more inclusive definitions suggest a higher incidence of disability (4-8%). The 2001 census found 21.91 million PWD (2.13%), while the 2002 NSS disability estimate is 1.8 per cent of the population.[1] The share of households estimated by NSS to have a disabled member was 8.4 per cent and 6.1 per cent in rural and urban areas respectively (though this share seems high given the number of disabled individuals and survey results on their household size) alternative estimates from a variety of sources suggest that the actual prevalence of disability in India could be easily around 400 million people, and as high as 80-90 million if more inclusion definitions of mental illness and mental retard ness in particular were used.[2] (the number is expected to rise with the reveling of census 2001 data because it has included 8 variety of disabilities, which was only 5 as parameter during 2001 census) The budget allocation goes according to the number of the group therefore at the formulation of policy planning, discrimination starts against the disable community. According to 2011 census, Indian population constitutes 17.50 per cent of the global population. It is an open secret that there are many basic necessities which is basic but all are not available in our country. India possesses a large number of poor people and it is a fact that South Asia where India shares two third of population and economy and everything which matter's, constitutes 50 per cent of the global poverty. Poverty itself is a great facilitator of disability and deprives the people with disability from the aspirations of a dignified life. Being a democratic country, India needs to guide by the cardinal principles of welfare state. It insists on the welfare of all with special care of the deprived sector. Disability sector has been deprived by twin counts from the governmental sector first at the level of the recognition of their number. They are no less than 10 per cent of the overall population. But governmental assertion those are only 2-3 per cent of the global population therefore allocation of the resources follows this dictate and deprives the community form their genuine aspiration to avail a dignified life. The 11th Five Year Plan (2007-12) is in progress and it has been stressed that the motto of 11th plan will be Inclusive Growth. Now the billion dollar question is that how it is possible not to accommodate one of the most deprived sectors of the society into the mainstreaming process of development.

The prevalence of rampant poverty is itself a great destroyer of justice based society. According to Arjun Sengupta (International Expert on Extreme Poverty and Human Rights and former Chairman, National Commission for Enterprises in the Unorganized Sector, Government of India) who is known expert of poverty at the global level poverty, especially extreme poverty, is the worst form of degradation of human dignity; a condition of absence of the most basic human rights.[3] However eradication of poverty has been an integral part of the campaign of the international human rights regime. Attempts are being made through United Nations and other international platform to abolish poverty by 2015. The UN has taken the consent of an absolute number of countries through United Nations Millennium Goals and poverty as an agenda of these goals to be achieved by 2015. It is just few years ahead and many governments have expressed their incapability to meet with the desired goals. Although governments and other concerned agencies have carried out gamut of efforts to eradicate poverty and ensure the basic necessities of the human being under which they could avail the basic dignity of their life. Many formulations have been evolved to cope with the challenges. But one of the best among them is the idea of capacity building propelled by Amartya Sen. Capacity according to Sen is "the opportunity to achieve valuable combinations of human functionaries; what a person is able to do or be".[4] In other words, the capability approach covers both the identification of the objectives of the substantive variables reflecting the freedom of people to be or to do what they want to be or do ; and also the methods of achieving these objectives, and choosing the instruments that are appropriate to each of those objectives. The way these instruments are to be used maintaining full accountability in a participatory framework is just as important as identifying the objectives. Capability as interpreted by Sen is equivalent to freedom to be or to do an individual values. Development, which has been described as an expansion of capabilities, has been captured by Sen in his *Development as Freedom*.[5] Poverty in that framework has been described as a severe deprivation of capability or lack of freedoms. Therefore development has given a new twist at the international level as a wider mechanism for the removal of human curse including poverty. In 1988, the UN has approved the Right to Development as an integral part of the international framework and an absolute number of countries have been its signatories. Earlier only civil and political rights were part and parcel of the framework of universally accepted rights but after the passage of this declaration it is the moral duty of the member state of the UN system to implement social and economic rights also as important instruments of rights.

These mechanisms are important for the resolution of the vicious circle of poverty and disability around the globe in general but for the Indian context in particular. The 2011 census data has already revealed that Indian population has grown to 121 crore. The level of poverty has also gone up. The poor people of India constitute more population than entire American population. As already stated that poverty is itself a great facilitator of disability and could be mitigated only through better employment opportunities for the poor in general and disable community in particular. The NSSO data 2002 also revealed the fact that majority of disability prevalence is within the poor groups. Without brining poor people is general and disable community in particular into the mainstreaming process of development, we could not achieve our much desired goal of sustainable development. Many international economic schools of thought have predicted that India will be within top three global economies by 2030. All important indicator of our development is growing. 2011 census data also supports this thesis. But the prevalence of acute poverty within the disable community is a matter of severe concern. It is the duty of all concern including the government and civil-society to take some crucial measures to contain this menace, which suppress the genuine aspirations of one of the most important deprived sectors of the society. Needless to say that much legislation has been enacted to cope with the challenges. But in India we know that implementation of any legislation has remained extremely weak due to variety of factors and it is the case with the implementation of disable friendly legislation too. With the ongoing pace of globalization, our corporate sector is mushrooming in a massive way. They need to impart philanthropy to correct the situation of the disable community. Merely governmental efforts are not enough because of the enormity of the problem. Our disable population is more than entire population of county like France. The corrective measures requires huge investments from all concerned including the government and the private sector and the notion of public-private partnership needs to be incorporated within this arena to harness the maximum benefits for the people with disability.

Eleventh five year plan is in progress and it was announced that 11th plan (2007-12) will be insisting on inclusive growth. According to the Approach Paper of the 11th plan "The 11th plan provides an opportunity to restructure policies to achieve a new vision of growth that would be much more broad based and inclusive, bringing about a faster reduction in poverty and helping bridge the divides that are currently the focus of so much attention. The first step in this direction was initiated in the middle of the Tenth Plan based on the National Common Minimum Programme adopted by the government. This step must be further strengthened and consolidated into a strategy for the 11th plan."[6]

The prevailing situation indicates that if India has to be poverty free country, if India has to be human rights friendly country then we have only one alternative in this regard and that is economic empowerment of the people with disability. As we have already discussed the matter that majority of disable people are able to work. But the question is we have already rampant unemployment for all despite the fact that our economy has been propelled in recent years and bound to keep the pace in future too. Disable people also have significantly lower employment rates than average, and this gap has been increasing over the last many years. The large majority of people with disability in India are capable of productive work. According to 2007 World Bank study the employment rate of the disabled population is lower (about 60 percent on average) than the general population, with the gap widening in the 1990.[7] Controlling the other factors, having a disability reduces the probability of being employed by for over 30 per cent for males in rural Uttar Pradesh and Tamil Nadu, though the effect is lower for women. However, those in rural areas and the better educated [those with post-graduate or vocational training] have relatively better prospects for employment relative to other disabled people. People with certain type of disabilities, e.g. hearing, speech and locomoter disabilities, and those with disability since birth also have better chances of getting a job. Mental illness and particularly mental retard ness have a strong negative impact on the probability of being employed, even in cases where such disabilities are not severe. The presence of a disable member also has impact on the labour supply of other adult household members. Around 45 per cent of households in UP and TN with a PWD report an adult missing work to care for PWD member, the bulk of these every day and on average for 205 hours. However, other adult men are more likely to be working in households with disable members, due to the need to compensate for lost income.[8] For the realization of the dream of India being a sustainable developed country we need to utilize the workforce potential of the disable community. It will take multi-dimensional approach for disable community to realize their full individual potential and to maximize their social and economic contribution to the society. Strengthening preventive and curative health care services, ensuring inclusion in education and increasing the participation of disabled in the workplace will be essential. The government of India has however initiated number of welfare schemes for the all round development of the disabled community but its implementation is prevented by corruption, lack of will power and bad governance. According to the World Bank study "India's implementation capacity is generally weak in a number pf areas of service delivery which are most critical to improving the situation of the people with disability, and it is not realistic to expect that all the actions needed by many public and non-public actors can be taken all at once. It is important therefore to decide the most critical interventions and get the basic rights first."[9]

The wider spectrum of disability movement in our country has been successful to aware the top brass of the system but the real issue has not been addressed yet. The awareness campaign has also remained confined to urban sectors and vast rural sectors remain aloof from this process. Although 2011 census data has come with certain positive indicators but rural sector still remains at the receiving end and we are aware the fact that still two-third population of our country lives in the rural sector. Therefore it is of utmost requirement to upgrade the life standard of the rural masses and in broader terms make their life self-dependent. We need to enhance the capacity building approach to people with disability. We have to break the vicious circle of poverty from their life and for that purpose we have to provide better employment opportunities to the people with disability. We have to provide some professional training also to them which could equip them to start even self made employment activities. It has been accepted by the UN and other prestigious international agencies that better employment opportunities could ensure the well being of the people. For the people with disability it is more correct. If we have to migrate their woes, than we have to provide better employment opportunities to them. It will not protect their life but encourage them to provide basic education to their next generation. In this situation their next generation will be enable to maximization of their possibilities. This process will enhance their standard of life and ensure for next generation.

We need to understand that the problem of disability in India has different context from their western counterpart. Still people with disability don't have basic amenities but in the western world they are already enjoying these basic rights and advocating to their next generation rights therefore we need to ensure for their basic rights first. In this context, employment has to play a vital role and we need to facilitate this process. Through accommodating their genuine requirements we could be able to play a facilitator role.

Our former President Kalam sahib kept reminding that India need to be a strong one within next couple of years. Many top guns of the international economics have also predicted this. We are doing well in all directions. But we need to upgrade the life standard to the people with disabilities. A democratic country must be known for the care it is imparting for their deprived citizens and needless to say that people with disability are one of the most deprived sectors of our society. India could not ensure sustainable development till it will not incorporate people with disability into the mainstreaming process of development. The process has already begun but we need to keep the momentum. We need to keep in our mind that people with disability are asking their parity with the able people, they are not asking for any charity. Being a democratic society we need to provide these elementary rights to people with disabilities. The articles included in this book deals with all pertinent issues related to the wider spectrum of the cause.

REFERENCES

1. Significantly, the two differ notably on the composition of the disabled population by type of disability. The difference are in part explained by different disability definitions in NSS and census.
2. See GoI/WHO and Dandona et al (2004) on visual and Gururaj and Issac [2005] on mental impairments.
3. Sengupta, Arjun, A Right Based Approach to Removing Poverty; Eradicating Poverty as Realizing Human Rights. *Indian Journal of Human Development,* Vol. 1, No. 1, 2007, p. 55.
4. Sen, Amartya, " Human Rights and Capabilities", *Journal of Human Development,* Vol. 6, No. 2, 2005, p. 153.
5. Sen, *Poverty as Capability, Development as Freedom,* Chapter, IV, Oxford University Press, 1999.
6. Towards Faster and More Inclusive Growth; An Approach to the 11th Five Year Plan, Planning Commission, Government of India, New Delhi, 2006.
7. It is important not to attribute these differentials entirely or automatically to discrimination, as many factors are at play, including lower than average educational levels and the nature of some disabilities. However, analysis in the report finds a significant unexplained element in employment participation probabilities. (See Chapter Five of the World Bank Report; 'People with Disabilities in India: From Commitments to Outcomes,' The World Bank, South Asia Region, 2007.)
8. World Bank Report, 'People with Disabilities in India: From Commitments to Outcomes,' The World Bank, South Asia Region, New Delhi, 2007, p. 13.
9. Ibid, p. 11.

PART I

DISABILITY PERSPECTIVES

1

Disability, Poverty and Sustainable Development: A New Outlook

Pankaj Sreshakar

What is Disability?

Defining disability is complex and controversial. Though arising from physical or intellectual impairment, disability has social implications as well as health ones. A full understanding of disability recognizes that it has a powerful human rights dimension and is often associated with social exclusion and increased exposure and vulnerability to poverty. Disability is the outcome of complex interactions between the functional limitations arising from a person's physical, intellectual, or mental condition and the social and physical environment. It has multiple dimensions and is far more than an individual health or medical problem. On this basis, the working definition of disability adopted in this paper is 'long-term impairment leading to social and economic disadvantages, denial of rights, and limited opportunities to play an equal part in the life of the community'.

Poverty: A Cause and Consequence

Poverty is both a cause and consequence of disability. Poverty and disability reinforce each other, contributing to increased vulnerability and exclusion. The majority of people with disabilities find their situation affects their chances of going to school, working for a living, enjoying family life, and participating as equals in social life. It is estimated that only 2 per cent of people with disabilities in developing countries have access to rehabilitation and appropriate basic services.

Poor nutrition, dangerous working and living conditions, limited access to vaccination programmes, and to health and maternity care, poor hygiene, bad sanitation, inadequate information about the causes of impairments, war and conflict, and natural disasters all cause disability. Many of these causes are preventable. According to estimates by the World Health Organisation (WHO), as many as 20 million women a year suffer disability and long-term complications as a result of pregnancy and childbirth. The most common causes of motor disability are injuries from accidents on the road, at home, or the workplace; war and violence, including landmines; birth trauma; and infectious diseases such as polio and leprosy. Children are often disabled as a result of malnutrition. In turn, disability exacerbates poverty, by increasing isolation and economic strain, not just for the individual but often for the affected family as well. Children with disabilities are more likely to die young, or be neglected, malnourished and poor. People with disabilities who are denied education is then unable to find employment, driving them more deeply into poverty. Breaking out of the vicious cycle of poverty and disability becomes more and more difficult. The result of the cycle of poverty and disability is that people with disabilities are usually amongst the poorest of the poor and their literacy rates are considerably lower than the rest of the population. Women with disabilities suffer a double discrimination, both on the grounds of gender and of impairment; their literacy rates are lower than their male counterparts. Recent UNESCO studies have suggested that only 1-2 per cent of children with disabilities in developing countries receive an education. Boys with disabilities attend school more frequently than girls with disabilities. Studies show that women with disabilities are twice to three times more likely to be victims of physical and sexual abuse than women with no disabilities. Their access to reproductive health care is minimal and as a result they suffer greater vulnerability to reproductive health problems. There is a lack of awareness regarding women with disabilities and reproductive health needs. More often than not, it is assumed that they do not form part of the target groups because being disabled is associated with being sexless.

As many as 50 per cent of disabilities are preventable and directly linked to poverty. For example, the WHO currently estimates that worldwide there are 1.5 million blind children, mainly in Africa and Asia. In developing countries up to 70 per cent of blindness in children is either preventable or treatable. The WHO also estimates that around 50 per cent of disabling hearing impairment is also preventable. In 1995 this affected a total of 120 million people worldwide.

Differential Needs

The needs of people with disabilities differ widely. Children, older people, women, indigenous people, refugees and displaced persons, minorities, and mentally-ill people may all experience disability differently. Some may suffer a multiple disadvantage as a result of their wider social or economic status. Even within these categories needs can differ widely, for example between richer and poorer women. The consequences are particularly severe for women with disabilities who are also subject to social, cultural and economic disadvantages due to gender discrimination. Moreover, a woman may become disabled due to an abuse of her rights. It is estimated that over 100 million girls and women in more than 28 countries in Africa alone are disabled as a result of female genital mutilation. The physical and psychological consequences of these practices range from mobility difficulties, impaired sexual function and infertility because of infection, to an increased risk of HIV infection.

In many developing countries women are assigned a low status, socially, economically and politically. This is accentuated when disability occurs. Girls and women with disabilities are left marginalized, neglected and are often considered a burden. Children are another vulnerable group. Mortality for children with disabilities may be as high as 80 per cent in countries where under-five mortality as a whole has decreased to below 20 per cent. In certain cases there seems to be a 'weeding out' of children with disabilities, the 'missing children'. Mental illness imposes a heavy burden in terms of human suffering, stigmatisation of the mentally ill and their families, and direct and indirect economic costs. The future burden is likely to grow over time as a result of an increasing and ageing global population, and increasing stresses resulting from social problems and unrest, including violence, conflict, and natural and other disasters.

Development is Linked with Poverty

In developing countries the proportion of people in income poverty by the $1-a-day measure declined from 34 per cent to 32 per cent in 1987-93, but the number of income poor people increased from 1.2 billion to 1.3 billion. The share of poor people declined rather slowly in east and south Asia, and in Sub-Saharan Africa and Latin America and the Caribbean it even increased. In 1993 South Asia was home to two fifths of the world's poor people, and East Asia and South East Asia and Pacific to a third.

And Poverty is linked to Human Development

Housing is fundamental to the formation of individual capabilities and to family and communities ties but more than a billion people in developing countries live without adequate shelter or inacceptable housing. At least 600 million people live in dwellings that threaten their health and lives. The most extreme housing deprivation is to have no home, and worldwide estimated 100 millions are homeless. Children are worst affected. In Brazil more than 2 lakh children spend their lives on the streets.

Simply put a quarter of the world's population lives in the poverty. In a global economy of $25 trillion this is a scandal—reflecting shameful inequalities and inexcusable failures of national and international policy.

So reference to developing countries must always be based on an understanding that the term include the most impoverished and deprived people in the world.

Poverty and Access to Information

The UNDP report focuses not just on poverty but on how poverty limits human choices and opportunities. Critical dimensions of human poverty... are lack of political freedom, inability to participate in the decision making, lack of personal security, inability to participate in life of community and threats to sustainability and intergenerational equity. Poverty also means a short life, lack of basic education and limited or no access to Public and Private Resources. One conclusion of the UNDP is that the face of Poverty is rapidly changing and the poverty trap may be inescapable.

> Today a poor person is more likely to be African, to be a child or a women or an elderly person in an urban area, to be landless, to live in an environmentally fragile area and to be a refugee or a displaced person....

Progress in reducing human and income poverty is marked by discontinuity and unevenness. The resulting disparity and the remaining backlog create and recreate human poverty, a continuing and non perpetuating process that the poor constantly struggle to overcome. Throughout the report, the UNDP stressed the importance of participating not only in combating poverty, but also in recording poverty.

> In constructing any index of poverty such as Human Poverty Index in this report the selection and the weights have to be explicitly stated and clarified so that the public scrutiny can occur. It is very important that the standards to be used are not determined on a top down basis, but are open to—if possible; emerge from a participatory, democratic process.

The guiding principles of our development process have been to ensure a decent standard of life to all. Yet, the results so far fall far short of desired goals. One third of our people continue to suffer from all forms of deprivation. The reasons may largely be attributed to the lack of people's participation in designing and implementation of poverty alleviation programmes and corruption. People's participation in decision making process is essence of democracy. Right based approach provides legal guarantee for realizing entitlements and ensures empowerment of people. Access to Information provides a framework for promoting Citizen-Government participation in development process.

The importance of Access to Information in Growth and Development

The UNDP emphasized the need to empower the ordinary person and ensure participation in the process that effect daily life.

A strategy for poverty eradication must focus not only on what need to be done but also on how to ensure that the action is taken, this requires such fundamental reforms as promoting political participation by all, ensuring accountability and transparency in government preventing the criminalization of politics, promoting free flow of information and freedom of press, and ensuring a strong role for community groups and NGOs in policy making and legislative decision making. Empowerment and participation will help to ensure the involvement of ordinary people in decision that affect their lives and enable them to build their strengths and assets. Uninformed people are clearly unable to participate fully in the political process. People who have access to information and who understand how to use that information in both the political and legal processes become empowered.

Such has been the case for 30,000 citizens of Ecuador who are taking a class action suit in New York against Texaco, a major Multinational Oil Corporation. Information is crucial in enabling people to make sound decision about their lives. Empowering people requires political commitments to policies that allow poor people to become less vulnerable. Access to Information is a key. The UNDP report noted that the economic resources to address poverty are not lacking—it is political will to tackle poverty head-on that is missing. Poor people must be visible on the political map if their interests are to be advanced. With access to information poor people can begin to organize themselves for collective action to influence the decisions affecting their lives. The culture of secrecy breeds corruption, which results in lower investments due to misuse of power and diversion of funds for private purposes.

- The Transparency International (TI) has reported that perceived corruption in India has declined.
- The corruption reduction score of 3.4 (out of 10) in 2008, after an initial rise of 3.5 in 2007, compared to 2.99 in 2006, which indicate a decline in corruption to the extent of 15 per cent.
- According to the TI-CMS survey study 40 per cent of the respondents have reported decline in corruption.

Right to information is harnessed as a tool for promoting participatory development, strengthening democratic governance and facilitating effective delivery of socio-economic services. At least 20 per cent of the information seekers are BPL cardholder and disabled. They have sought to know the reasons as to why the services meant for them are not reaching them. The poor persons are increasingly involved in designing and implementation of poverty alleviation programmes.

The benefits of the government schemes hardly reached them due to inefficiency and corruption. The adoption of rights-based approach is significant to weed out corruption and to guarantee the reach of entitlements of poor persons. The poverty alleviation programmes are designed such that a citizen can observe and scrutinize the public activities.

An informed citizenry is putting desirable pressure on the concerned departments for effective implementation of flagship programmes like *Bharat Nirman,* which seeks to provide critical infrastructure like rural roads, electricity, water and sanitation for rural population. The trend in partnership between citizen and the Government indicate that RTI regime would help create solid infrastructure required for rapid poverty reduction.

Development Aid and Right to Know: The status of the recipients

Viewing economic resources at a global level, the UNDP has noted that commercial globalization may offer opportunities for reducing poverty, but only with careful management of these resources and more equitable distribution of benefits. Currently the least developed countries have 10 per cent of the world's people but only 0.3 per cent of world trade. This is half their shares of two decades ago. The enormous disparity between the world's "haves" and have-nots" is clear from the following figures:

> The share of the poorest 20 per cent of the world's people in global income now stands at a miserable 1.1 per cent down from 1.4 per cent in 1991 and 2.35 per cent in 1960. It continues to shrink and the ratio of the income of the top 20 per cent of that of the poorest 20 per cent rose from 30 to 1 in 1960, to 61 to 1 in 1991—and to startling new high of 78 to 1 in 1994.

The UNDP found that two factors contributing to these inequitable situations are:

> Average tariffs on Industrial country imports from the least developed countries are 30 per cent higher than the global average—Developing countries lose about $60 billion a year than agricultural subsidies and barriers to textile export in industrial nation.

According to the Report, International Aid has been declining. It should be increased and better directed by donors. Three major initiatives are suggested:

> More aid for the Sub-Saharan and other least developed countries, a shift in the use of aid away from expatriate technical assistance personnel and towards long term support for national capacity, a greater concentration of aid on countries demonstrating serious commitment to poverty reduction and human development.

With regard to reproductive health, failure to provide basic information and medical resources has had devastating effects:

An estimated 5 lakhs women die each year from avoidable pregnancy related causes, unsafe abortions cause the deaths of between 60000 and 2 lakhs women annually and result in long term ill health for at least 1 million others, AIDS has killed an estimated 2.5 million people and the rate of HIV infection is thought to have doubled between 1990 and 1993.

On the positive side, an information project of a Chinese Government and the United Nations Populations Fund is regarded as a breakthrough in removing coercion from family planning in China.

The financial resource to give effects to plans such as these, based on access to Information, are in the gift of the industrialize nations but decision on landing, spending, and borrowing are taken behind the closed doors of the World Bank and the IMF.

The Perspective of Freedom

It is not unusual for the couples to discuss the possibility of earning more money but a conversation on this subject from around the 8th century BC is of some special interest. As that conversation is recounted in Sanskrit Text *Brihadaranyaka Upanishada,* a woman named Maitreyee and her husband, Yajnavalkya proceed rapidly to a bigger issue of than the ways and the means of becoming more wealthy: *how far would wealth go to help them get what they want?* Maitreyee wonders whether it could be the case that "the whole earth full of wealth" were to belong just to her, she could achieve immortality through it. 'No', responds Yagyavalkya, "Like the life of rich people will be your life. But there is no hope of immortality by wealth." Maitreyee remarks, "What should I do with that by which I do not become immortal?"

Maitreyee's rhetorical question has been cited again and again in Indian religious philosophy to illustrate both the nature of human predicament and the limitations of the material world. The issue is not the ability of live forever on which Maitreyee—bless her soul—happened to concentrate, but the capability to live really long and to have a good life while alive—things that would be strongly valued and desired by nearly all of us. This is not because income and wealth are desirable for their own sake, but because typically, they are admirable general purpose means for having more freedom to lead the kind of lives we have reason to value.

The ends and means of development require examination and scrutiny for a fuller understanding of the development process; it is simply not adequate to take our basic objective just the maximization of income or wealth, which is as Aristotle noted, "merely useful and for the sake of something else." For the same reason, economic growth cannot sensibly be treated as an end in itself. Development has to be more concerned with enhancing the lives we lead and the freedoms we enjoy. Expanding the freedom that we have reason to value not only makes our lives richer and more unfettered, but also allows us to be fuller social persons, exercising our own volitions and interacting with—and influencing—the world in which we live.

Economists are sometimes criticized for concentrating too much on deficiency and too little on equity. There may be some ground for complaint here, but it must also be noted that inequality has received attention from economists from throughout the history of this discipline. If there is a reason to grumble, it rests more on relative importance that is attached, in much of economics, to inequality in a very narrow domain, viz., *income inequality.*

Empirically, the relationship between income inequality and inequality in other relevant spaces can be rather distant and contingent because of various economic influences other than income that affect inequalities in individual advantages and substantive freedoms. For example, in the higher mortality rates of African Americans vis-à-vis the much poorer Chinese, or Indians in Kerala, we see the influence of factors that run in the opposite direction to income inequality, and that involve public policy issues with strong economic components: the financing of health care and insurance, provision of public education, arrangements for local security and so on.

Despite the crucial role of incomes in the advantages enjoyed by different persons, the relationship between income and other resources, on the other hand, and other individual achievements and freedoms, on the other, is neither constant nor in any sense automatic and irresistible. The argument is sometimes made that income is homogeneous magnitude, whereas capabilities are diverse. This sharp contrast is not entirely correct, in the sense that any income evaluation hides internal diversities with some special—and often heroic—assumptions. The issue of public discussion and social participation is thus central to the making of policy in a democratic framework. The use of democratic prerogatives—both political liberties and civil rights—is a crucial part of the exercise of economic policy itself, in addition to other roles it may have. In a freedom oriented approach, the participatory freedoms cannot but central to public policy analysis.

Developing and strengthening a democratic system is an essential component of the process of development. The significance of democracy lies in three distinct virtues:

Its intrinsic importance,
Its instrumental contributions, and
Its constructive role in the creation of values and norms.

No evaluation of the democratic form of governance can be complete without considering each. Despite their limitations, political freedoms and civil rights are used effectively often enough.

The perspective of freedom has been used both in evaluative analysis for assessing change, and in the descriptive and predictive analysis in seeing freedom as a causally effective factor in generating rapid change. This diversity is not, however, a matter of regret. As William Cowper puts it:

Freedom has a thousand charms to show,
That slaves, howe'er contended, never know.

Development is indeed a momentous engagement with freedom's possibilities.

Right of Access to Media and Information Communication Technologies (ICTs)

International Standards

Article 19 of the Universal Declaration of Human Rights 1948, states that everyone has a right to, '... seek, receive and impart information and ideas through any media and regardless of frontiers.'

The ICCPR in Article 19 further expands this right recognizing that information can be received and imparted, 'orally, in writing or in print, in the form of art or through any media of [her/his] choice.'

The UN Special Rapporteur on Freedom of Opinion and Expression in his Annual Report, 1998 noted, '[T]he right to seek, receive and impart information imposes a positive obligation on States to ensure access to information, particularly with regard to information held by Government in all types of storage and retrieval systems... .'

Studies carried out in Asia, Europe and America suggest that disabled and non-disabled have similar media habits. Relevance of television, radio and newspapers is as significant in the lives of persons with disabilities as it is for the non-disabled population.

Rule 5 of the Standard Rules also calls on States to 'encourage the media, especially television, radio and newspapers, to make their services accessible' to persons with disabilities.

There is now a political will in many countries to ensure access to various forms of media and culture by persons with disabilities. New legal frameworks and standards are being developed to promote the concept of universal design and universal service. The telecommunication, broadcasting and information laws and regulations falling short of accessibility standards are being repealed or amended. The effort is towards creating systems independent of individual bias as a means to overcome the digital divide.

Telecommunication

The international efforts for setting universal standards in telecom, media and information processing in last ten years have gone a long way in ensuring access to media, information and culture by persons with disabilities. For instance, six different text telephone systems for the deaf and deaf blind came in use but with serious problems of compatibility, interoperability and limitations in international calling. Therefore, in 1997/98 the International Telecommunications Union (ITU) through Study Group T16 released three major recommendations:

- V.18 describes a multi-function text telephone, which can communicate with the wide variety of text telephones in use today;
- T.140 adds new facilities, which allow text communication using a very wide variety of alphabets such as Arabic, Cyrillic, Kanji etc. as well as Latin-based characters; and
- T.134 describes how these facilities are used in the multimedia communications systems defined by the ITU-T. (Gunnar Hellstrom, 1998)

After having completed work on V.18, T.140 and T.134, the ITU focused its attention on three new targets with the objective to:

- Establish an interoperability test for text telephones;
- To establish interworking between text conversation in different environments by adding to Recommendation H.246 on interworking between the different multimedia systems; and
- To establish a service description for multimedia conversation services, including text conversation and video with motion reproduction sufficient for sign language and lip reading.

The European Telecommunications Standards Institute (ETSI) has also produced three very significant deliverables that provide guidance to the designers of communication products and services. These include:

- ETR 029: Human Factors (HF); Access to telecommunications for people with special needs; Recommendations for improving and adapting telecommunication terminals and services for people with impairments (1991);
- ETR 116: Human Factors (HF); Human factors guidelines for ISDN Terminal equipment design; (1994); and
- ETR 166: Human Factors (HF); Evaluation of telephones for people with special needs; An evaluation method (1995).

Web Accessibility

In the last decade or so, Internet has brought about a radical shift in the paradigm of information dissemination, sharing and processing. Using Internet in a variety of information forms like plain/formatted text, pictures, audio and video can be presented to the users across the globe at a fast, reliable and extremely cost effective manner. While the variety in the forms of information makes the content aesthetically very appealing and easy to use, it also poses new challenges for people with disabilities.

Shapiro and Varian, authors of Information Rules: A Strategic Guide to the Network Economy, point out that 'today more than 60 percent of Internet traffic is to Web Sites, and of the Web traffic, almost three-fourths is images.' Therefore, information on the web loaded with graphics and images cause a serious threat to the freedom of information for those with sight impairment. Similarly, Web pages with a long list of hyperlinks crowded together could confuse a person with learning disabilities. Even people with hearing disabilities find it difficult to access the content of audio streaming and video clips posted on the Internet in the absence of captioning.

It is worth noting that Rule 5 of the Standard Rules also refers to 'new computerized information and service systems offered to the general public' and urges governments to ensure that they are 'made initially accessible or are adapted to be made accessible to persons with disabilities.'

In consonance with this requirement in the Standard Rules, a development worth noticing is the release of the 'Web Content Accessibility Guidelines 1.0' specification issued by World Wide Web Consortium (W3C) on May 5, 1999. This significant development provides a stable specification that has been reviewed and recommended by the W3C Membership as a tool for making web sites accessible. The specification contains fourteen guidelines which are general principles of accessible design. Each guideline is associated with one or more checkpoints describing how to apply that guideline to particular features of Web pages. An appendix to the guidelines, 'Checklist of Checkpoints for the Web Content Accessibility Guidelines 1.0' presents the checkpoints sorted by priority for easy reference.

Several worthwhile initiatives have been reported by the UN Secretary-General on the action taken to promote awareness and build national capacities for Internet accessibility. These efforts have been carried out in co-operation with Government, non-government and private bodies in various parts of the world. They are reflected in the Secretary General's Progress Report on implementation of the WPA to the fifty-fourth session of the General Assembly (1999; document A/54/388/Add.1) and the fifty-sixth session of the General Assembly (2001; document A/56/169) and to the thirty-ninth session of the Commission for Social Development (2001).

Media

The mass media has undergone rapid transformation by simulating major technological innovations such as electronics editing, publishing and through animated images and digitized production of TV programming. The computerized and communication-assisted publishing of the printed press has also contributed to this revolution. Interactive television and multimedia has opened up unprecedented opportunities for entertainment, education and commerce. If the rapidly developing media technologies are made available based on the principle of universal design, the media's capacity to break down traditional barriers to participation by disadvantaged groups such as the people with disabilities are enormous.

Towards this end, Biwako Millennium Framework encourages international organizations (e.g., International Telecommunication Union, International Organization for Standardization, World Trade Organization, World Wide Web Consortium, Motion Picture Engineering Group) responsible for international ICT standards to incorporate by 2004 accessibility standards for persons with disabilities in their international ICT standards.

Domestic Standards

The recognition of a distinct disability culture in countries of Europe and North America has been instrumental in promoting accessible media there. The situation in countries in Asia, Latin America and Africa is not so encouraging. There is a persistent indifference to the cultural identity of persons with disabilities and not much has been done to promote their participation in the mainstream cultural life. As a consequence the related laws in India, such as Information Technology Act, Prasar Bharati (Broadcasting Corporation of India) Act, 1990, and Telecom Regulatory Authority of India Act lack disability perspective.

The NHRC is alive to the fact that telecommunications, broadcasting and other systems of information are out of the reach of a vast majority of persons with disabilities due to their cost and standards of design and delivery. Hence, in January 2003 it recommended that Government of India and State Governments should elaborate and adopt a National/State policy on accessible infrastructure for persons with disabilities in order to ensure barrier free access to built environment, transport system, telecommunication, information and broadcasting and electronic public information facilities.

Broadcasting Norms

Prasar Bharati (Broadcasting Corporation of India) is the State supported broadcaster in India. This autonomous entity is regulated by the Prasar Bharati (Broadcasting Corporation of India) Act, 1990. While specifying the functions of Prasar Bharati the Act focuses on the interests of minority and weaker sections. Section 12(1) states the primary duty of the Corporation and Section 12(2) outlines the functions as follows:

(a) upholding the unity and integrity of the country and the values enshrined in the Constitution;
(b) safeguarding the citizen's right to be informed freely, truthfully and objectively on all matters of public interest, national or international, and presenting a fair and balanced flow of information including contrasting views without advocating any opinion or ideology of its own;
(c) paying special attention to the fields of education and spread of literacy, agriculture, rural development, environment, health and family welfare and science and technology;
(d) providing adequate coverage to the diverse cultures and languages of the various regions of the country by broadcasting appropriate programmes;
(e) providing appropriate coverage to sports and games so as to

encourage healthy competition and the spirit of sportsmanship;

(f) providing appropriate programmes keeping in view the special needs of the youth;

(g) informing and stimulating the national consciousness in regard to the status and problems of women and paying special attention to the upliftment of women;

(h) promoting social justice and combating exploitation, inequality and such evils as untouchability and advancing the welfare of the weaker sections of the society;

(i) safeguarding the rights of the working classes and advancing their welfare;

(j) serving the rural and weaker sections of the people and those residing in border regions, backward or remote areas;

(k) providing suitable programmes keeping in view the special needs of the minorities and tribal communities; and

(i) taking special steps to protect the interests of the children, the blind, the aged, the handicapped and other vulnerable Sections of the people (emphasis added).

Despite such a clear mandate, as indicated in clause l above, there are numerous constraints to access television programming by persons with disabilities. User Interface Standards, User Presentation Standards and Terminal Equipment Standards need to be developed and redefined so that all analogue and digital broadcasting services are delivered on the principle of universal design and accessibility norms. Towards this end, the NHRC has recommended formation of a multi sectoral task force comprising various

Ministries and autonomous bodies in the Government of India and including people with disabilities and universal design experts. Such a task force has been advised to identify areas of review, assessment, research and finally to come up with a National Accessible Infrastructure Policy and Plan.

It is interesting to note that in Section 12(2)(o) the Prasar Bharati Act provides for 'promoting research and development activities in order to ensure that radio and television broadcast technology are constantly updated.'

In Europe, Governments plan to provide much of their information and services via digital television. Therefore, incorporation of accessible features in the design of digital broadcasting and its delivery system has received considerable attention.

Rigorous media research initiatives from a disability perspective have been undertaken through a multidisciplinary approach with broadcasters, ICT companies, and academic and disability organizations working together. The studies of this nature generally analyse user's concerns, information and broadcasting laws, design of existing media products and their delivery mechanism and most often these researches offer design solution based on universal design principles and accessibility norms.

In a rapidly changing era of media technology, it becomes all the more important to encourage universal design principles. To accommodate the challenge of technology switchover, parallel changes in the related laws become imperative. UK presents a good case study in this regard where, in the year 1996, the government adopted a new Broadcasting Act. This coincided with broadcast technology switch from analogue to digital. The Act mandates broadcast of at least 10 per cent programmes with narration or verbal description of key visual elements of a programme. However, the Act does not contain any provision for audio description transmission and reception standards. Therefore, when digital terrestrial television started in the UK in November 1999, no provision was made for transmission of verbal description of visual elements because the digital terrestrial set top boxes were not configured to download audio description feature. As a result, the blind and elderly persons got deprived of the narrative video service, which would have allowed them full access to television.

Telecommunications

Like television, telephones play an equally important role in the lives of people with disabilities. When Alexander Graham Bell invented the telephone, he was attempting to convert speech into a visual representation to accommodate a greater choice of information modality for his wife who had a hearing loss. Unfortunately, Bell's invention failed to accommodate conversion of information from auditory to visual mode as intended. Instead, the long distance communication scenario got transformed completely, allowing communication in real time for persons who could hear. The intended benefits of telecommunication for the hearing impaired and deaf came about much later. The Teletypewriter (TTY) service that enabled communication for the deaf with other TTY users became available in the United States during the mid-70s. The Tele-relay service became the second milestone that widened the communication choice as through a relay centre the deaf callers could communicate with hearing persons. These technologies had their own limitations in terms of compatibility, interoperability and long distance calling. The International Telecommunications Union (ITU) has addressed all these issues and now norms for accessible telecom are available.

The development of videophones has benefited deaf and hard of hearing people beyond estimation. This means that deaf people now can use videophones to communicate in sign language in the same way as hearing people use telephones. In fact, recent improvements in the quality of pictures in the videophone are also an outcome of a disability concern, as sign language users demanded a faster and clearer image processing. After having completed its work on V.18, T.140 and T.134, the ITU focused on establishing a service description for multimedia conversation services, including text conversation and video with motion reproduction sufficient for sign language and lip reading.

Web Accessibility

In the last few years judicial, quasi-judicial and several administrative authorities have interpreted the anti discrimination provisions to uphold the right to access technology mediated information. The concept of access is very dynamic and disability has contributed to its further evolution. The following examples from the USA, Australia and the UK demonstrate how access is interpreted as a means to achieving non-discrimination in the information society.

In November 1999, the National Federation of the Blind filed a suit against America Online, Inc., charging that AOL's proprietary browser and Internet web site was inaccessible to consumers who are blind. In March 2000, a settlement was reached under Americans with Disabilities Act (ADA) between the Bank of America and the California Council of the Blind requiring to not only install 2500 talking ATMs in Florida and California, but also to ensure that its website and online banking services were accessible to people using screen readers.

The Attorney General of Connecticut, USA settled a complaint filed by National Federation of the Blind v/s four online tax filing services. As per this settlement, four online tax filing services listed on the web site of Revenue Department were modified to ensure that people who are blind can access the sites with effect from tax filing year 2000 in accordance with Americans with Disabilities Act. It is pertinent to mention here that Americans with Disabilities Act is a non-discrimination legislation.

By a reference dated 26 August 1999, the Attorney-General (Australia), inter alia, advised the Human Rights and Equal Opportunity Commission to examine the difficulties and restrictions faced by older Australians and those with a disability in achieving full and equal access to services utilizing new technologies and deriving full benefit from such technologies.

The Commission was further advised to conduct an audit of the accessibility of Australian government and business Internet sites, with reference to the Disability Discrimination Act and relevant Australian and International guidelines.

The part three of the Disability Discrimination Act, 1995 of the UK requires providers of goods, facilities and services to make them accessible to people with impairments. This provision has been interpreted to emphasize that 'Unlawful discrimination occurs when a service provider discriminates, by doing one of the following:

- Refusing to serve a disabled person;
- Offering a disabled person a lower standard of service;
- Offering a disabled person less favourable terms; and
- Failing to make alterations to a service or facility, which makes it impossible, or unreasonably difficult, for a disabled person to use.'

With the exception of intervention by the NHRC recommending

the Government to constitute a multi-sectoral taskforce to ensure access on equal basis to people with disabilities, no other example of a legally mandated entity taking initiative to modify ICT related laws can be found in India. It is ironical that India is an IT leader but its IT laws remain limited in their purpose and scope with no concern for access to public or private sites for persons with disabilities; and all this when the World Summit of Information Society (WSIS) is galvanizing a dynamic set of principles that would set the stage for a knowledge based information society in which access without discrimination would be ensured for all.

Whether nurturing of cultures, popularization of science or influencing public opinion, the media is likely to play a more significant role than ever before. Therefore, media's importance in mainstreaming disability has increased manifold. The academics, researchers, and the disability rights' activists need to take a hard look on the laws and regulations that govern media, and information technology services with a view to suggesting improvements from a disability standpoint.

Concluding Remarks: Tasks Ahead

A major challenge is to develop capacities for access to information for the disabled population. The capacities of both the public authorities (i.e. the duty-bearers) and the citizens (i.e. the claim holders) may have to be enhanced. The Government has to develop a comprehensive Information Management System for storage and retrieval of data and information that may be shared with anyone who seeks it. At the moment awareness level among the disabled poor is less than 10 per cent, which is a major obstacle in reaping the benefits of Civil Rights for securing entitlements to the poor. Therefore, one has to create mass awareness among the poor disabled people. The Government of the day has to adopt multimedia approach to educate and train the disadvantaged class as to how to decide and select what information should be sought for and that from where and how?

Promotion of information literacy and democratization of knowledge resources, are vital for people's empowerment and for ensuring the reach of entitlements to the beneficiaries as well as for equalizing opportunities for sharing the benefits of development.

The Union Cabinet approved the National e-Governance Plan (NeGP) in May, 2006 which adopted the vision of making "all government services accessible to the common man in his locality, through common service delivery outlets and ensure efficiency, transparency and reliability of such services at affordable costs to realize the basic needs of the common man".

The reference to the common man in the vision brings to mind the 70 percent of the country's population of 1.1 billion that lives in its villages. Any programme seeking to extend electronic services through a single window to the citizenry will only be meaningful if it has a clear game plan for addressing this segment. A key component of the game plan for extending access under NeGP is the Common Services Centres (CSC) scheme, implemented by the Department of Information Technology, GoI. The scheme envisages creation of a network of over 100,000 CSCs as common access points throughout the country on a PPP basis. These CSCs would function as outlets for Government and private services. A typical CSC (one for every six villages) would be a Broadband and Internet-enabled Kiosk, which would be managed by a trained Village Level Entrepreneur providing "assisted access" to the villager. The kiosk would have a PC along with basic support equipment like Printer, Scanner, UPS, etc. As on date (October 2008), around 18,000 CSCs have already been set up on the ground. 25 States are at an advanced stage of activity for setting up a total 87,419 CSCs, with the remaining having registered significant progress in their preparatory work.

Another key component linking the Government with the citizen is the State Wide Area Network (SWAN) that seeks to connect Govt. offices across all levels (from the State Headquarters to Block level through District/Sub-Division Headquarters) with a minimum of 2 Mbps connectivity. A third infrastructure pillar is the State Data Centre that comprises the basic computing infrastructure to be shared across Government Departments/offices at the State level. A Capacity Building Scheme has also been approved early this year for creating human resource capacities at the State level for conceptualization and management of IT infrastructure and projects. The above four key components together have a financial outlay of Rs 11,000 crores and are expected to be fully operational in most states by June, 2009.

States have been encouraged to leverage this core infrastructure and provide single window access for all Govt. services over the Internet by creating State Portals that would be accessible from the CSCs and would enable citizens to access forms and submit various applications electronically through e-Forms. Each States would also establish a "State Service Delivery Gateway" that would route all the e-Forms filed from CSCs to respective field offices connected over the SWAN. Such a delivery mechanism will provide the citizens electronic acknowledgement of application submission and subsequent tracking of the status of the application.

While the above approach takes care of the front-end access provision for citizens, there is a concomitant need for the large number of Government departments at Central, State and local Government levels to redesign their back-end processes to enable service delivery to citizens along pre-defined standards. The NeGP has accordingly listed out a set of 27 Mission Mode Projects spanning all tiers of the Government. Each Project will need to define services that would be delivered to citizens and businesses at predefined service levels. Departments would need to focus on carrying out necessary procedural and legal reforms to enable achievement of project objectives in terms of service delivery to citizens. One of these MMPs is the e-district project that seeks to enable 10 high volume services within each district for electronic delivery. Six of the ten services have been mandated nationally, while four are left to each state to choose. Of the six centrally mandated services under the e-district scheme, one is RTI services. Pilot projects under the e-district MMP are currently under implementation in 40 districts.

The ultimate objective would be to have an end-to-end electronic processing of citizens' requests using systems housed at the SDCs delivering services over the network/gateway to the CSCs. However, recognizing the complexity and time involved in fully computerizing backend operations within multiple Govt. departments, the States have been advised to focus initially on provision of electronic front ends through the CSCs with the backend processing continuing in the manual mode. As an immediate step, States/UTs have been advised to convert all existing manual forms into e-Forms for electronic submission over the State Portal. Also, while implementing the suggested approach, States have been advised to consider Departments delivering high volume services, such as those delivered from the main district headquarters and subordinates offices.

Clearly, the task at hand is mammoth by any standards—one that requires us to marry the hard information technology skills with softer skills requiring appreciation of simple human needs and concerns and "healing the pain points" in government—citizen interfaces.

REFERENCES

1. Reinventing Public Service Delivery in India: Selected Case Studies, Edited by Vikram K Chand, World Bank, Sage Publication (2006).
2. Development As Freedom by Amartya Sen, Oxford India Press (2000).
3. Right To Information—Law—Policy—Practice by Rodney D Ryder, Wadhwa Nagpur (2006).
4. Human Development Report 2005 by Oxford University Press.
5. Disability, Poverty and Development: A report by DFID (1997).
6. Report of NHRC, Government of India (2006).
7. National Portal of India, http://india.gov.in

2

Definitional and Enumeration Inconsistencies: A case for Review Differently Abled Population:

Bhupinder Zutshi

Inconsistencies of estimating the magnitude of Differently Abled population in India poses serious difficulties in providing appropriate social, psychological, medical and economic supportive environment to the disabled persons. Disability prevalence estimates often differ across and within countries. Developed countries have enumerated higher disability rates as compared to developing countries due to definitional variations, under counting and reporting errors due to technically untrained enumerator, while conducting enumerations in developing countries. Several types of disabilities are invisible and can be identified only after thorough probing by experienced and trained enumerators. Unfortunately the system of enumeration in India is faulty as experienced and trained enumerator's do not conduct such census, hence a significant proportion of disabled people are left out of enumeration. Moreover the social stigma attached to disability, lower education and awareness level of respondents also makes actual disabled population invisible as disability is usually self-reported. This is clearly reflected by variations in the estimated disabled population even by the two major government sources of Census Operations and NSSO. According to the 58th round of the National Sample Survey (NSSO-2002), there were 18.5 million persons with disabilities in 2002 as compared to 21.9 million reported disabled persons by the Census of 2001. This translates to a 20 percent difference in the prevalence estimate rates. Owing to the inconsistency of data enumeration for disabled persons, the policy prescriptions have been faulty especially providing appropriate services, budget allocations and other facilities. In the light of such discrepancies in estimating the actual magnitude of differently abled persons, it is important to examine the appropriate definition of disability measurements across global perspective.

According to various NSSO surveys, there were 13.67 million disabled persons in 1981, 16.36 million disabled persons in 1991 (who were having at least one or more of the four types of disabilities viz., locomotor, visual, hearing and speech) and 18.49 million disabled persons in 2002. The NSSO survey 58th Round in 2002, covered mental disability in addition to the above stated four disabilities. The 2001 census recorded 21.91 million people with disability (2.13 per cent of the total population). About 10.63 per cent of the disabled persons suffered from more than one type of disabilities. The Census of India-2001 depicted that 58 percent differently abled were males and 42 percent were females. Hence disability was more prevalent among males.

Differently Abled Population: Enumeration Inconsistency in India

The history of collecting census in India dates back to 1871, when first census was conducted under the British rule. The questionnaire of 1872, called the 'House Register' included questions not only on the physically disabled but also the intellectually disabled persons and persons affected by leprosy. However this practice was discontinued after the 1931 census.

The comeback of disability census in 1981, after a gap of nearly 50 years, was at an opportune time as the United Nations had declared the year as the 'International Year of the Disabled'. The question in the census of 1981, asked people, if any person in the households were, totally blind, totally crippled and/or totally disabled. Enumerators were not appropriately trained to collect this sensitive information. As was expected, the total numbers of disabled persons recorded at the national level were only 0.16 percent of the total enumerated population. Only 1,118,948 disabled persons from rural areas and 149,547 disabled persons from urban areas were recorded in 1981 census, which was contrary to several estimated figures given by different government and NGOs sources. The data of 1981 census for disabled persons created a lot of confusion about the actual magnitude of disabled persons in India. Ministry of Social Welfare requested the National Sample Survey Organization (NSSO) to devote 37th Round in 1981, especially for collecting data on disability, to clear the air of confusion created by the census data. Subsequently because of the inadequacies of data collection for disabled persons in 1981 the census discontinued disability question again in 1991 Census. Instead NSSO round 47th in 1991 was also devoted to gather information for disabled population from selected sample areas.

The decade of 1990-2000 witnessed intense lobbying and pressure mounted from civil society organizations throughout the country for prevention, protection and rehabilitation of disabled persons, as it was considered as a rights issue instead of welfare measure. This pressure culminated into passing of the Prevention of Disability Act (PWD Act, 1995) in the Indian parliament for providing equal opportunities to disabled persons. Intense lobbying and pressure also resulted in inclusion of a question on disability in the Census 2001, to ascertain the magnitude and types of disability in India. Separate questions on disability were included in the census 2001. Emphasis was given to provide appropriate training to the enumerators to record the disabled people correctly in 2001 Census. Subsequently NSSO devoted 58th round in 2002 for collecting information on disabled persons to supplement the data recorded in 2001 census as well as for helping policy makers to draw comparative picture on disability in continuation to data collected in the NSSO rounds of 1981 and 1991.

Estimates of the number of disabled persons in India vary a great deal because of varying definitions adopted by different enumerating agencies, sources of data, the methodology used for data collection and the extent of use of scientific instruments in identifying and measuring the degree of disability. The National Sample Survey Organisation (NSSO) conducted three countrywide sample surveys in 1981, 1991 and 2002 for measuring the extent and types of disabled persons in India.

It is important to try and understand the differences in prevalence estimates from the Census of India-2001 and the 58th round of the NSSO survey conducted in 2002. The factors that contribute to the differences between the two sources include different sampling designs, understanding of disability definition perceptions and methods adopted for enumeration. The Census and the NSSO have different sampling design. The Census is an enumeration of the entire population of India while the NSSO has a nationally representative stratified sample across appropriately selected NSSO regions. In both sources, disability was self-reported as enumerators were not trained to identify and diagnose disability parameters. Therefore there is tendency to under report the cases of disability especially those cases which cannot be observed and are hidden. Moreover different definitions of overall disability and various disability types may have contributed to differences in estimates of disabled population in general and among different types of disabled person in particular.

The Census of 2001 does not have a general definition of disability. Instead, a question on type of disability was included in the population enumeration section as follows: "If the person is physically/mentally disabled, give appropriate code number from the list below, five codes were specified for this purpose." These codes were, "disability in seeing, in Speech, in hearing, in movement, mental." The Census thus has a functional limitation question, which prompts respondents to report their type of functional limitation (e.g., in seeing, hearing only and hinders several other types of disabilities which require specialized probing).

Although the question on disability has been vastly enlarged in Census 2011, yet it suffers from the conceptual understanding of functional disability to social exclusion and psychological disability. In comparison to the 5 Codes in Census 2001, 8 Codes have been provided in the Census 2011. In addition to the existing 5 types of functional disabilities recorded in 2001, three new codes were introduced in the Census 2011. These three new codes were "Mental Retardation, Mental Illness and any other and Multiple Disability". These questions and the instructions were finalized after extensive deliberations with civil society organizations and ministry of Social Justice and Empowerment. Respondents with multiple disabilities would now be able to report up to 3 disabilities for the first time.

Similarly in the case of NSSO, a person is considered disabled "if the person has restrictions or lack of abilities to perform an activity in the manner or within the range considered normal for a human being". Disability is thus defined as an activity limitation even in the NSSO and considers functional parameters rather than socio-psychological aspects. Thus a large number of disabled described in the global perspective are excluded from the enumeration due to technical grounds. Therefore large scale under-reporting of magnitude of disabled population have been reported both by Census 2001 report as well as by the NSSO-2002 report. There is possibility that this under reporting will continue even in 2011 Census, although the enumeration methodology has improved with better trained enumeration staff. This under reporting has severe policy implications as required services, budget allocations and incentives do not match with the actual magnitude of differently abled population.

In both Census and NSSO sources, persons who report being disabled are asked about their limitation types (mental, locomotor, visual, hearing, speech), which have been now expanded to three more disability types in 2011. Despite similar sequence in the identification of disability types, there are also tremendous variations in prevalence estimates of types of disability across the two data sources. As in the case of visual disability higher proportion was recorded by the Census (50 percent) as compared to only (15.3 percent) by the NSSO. For visual disability, the Census includes persons, who have blurred vision and have had no occasion to test their vision. It thus includes persons who may be able to see with spectacles. In contrast, the NSSO does not consider whether or not a person's vision has been tested and focuses on the ability to perform tasks requiring visual acuity.

Similarly in the case of hearing disability the Census recorded lower proportion of hearing disabled persons (5.8 percent) as compared to the NSSO data, which recorded (16.6 percent) hearing disabled. For hearing disability, persons who can hear only with one ear are counted as disabled in the Census, while they are considered as non disabled in the NSSO. In addition, the Census refers to hearing ability when the person uses hearing aid (if at all) while the NSSO refers to a person's hearing ability without the use of hearing aid.

Speech disabled proportion of population recorded by the Census-2001 was lower (7.5 percent) as compared to (11.7 percent) in the NSSO data 2002. The NSSO has a broader definition of speech disability than the Census. According to the NSSO, persons who cannot speak, speak limited words or with loss of voice, or with stammering voice are classified as being speech disabled. While in the Census, Speech disability covers persons who are dumb, or who cannot be understood. A person who stammers but whose speech is comprehensible is not considered as speech disabled according to the Census definition.

Again Locomotor disabled proportion of disabled population was lower as per the Census 2001 data (27.9 percent) as compared to (57.5 percent) recorded by the NSSO-2002. The NSSO has a broader definition related to locomotor disability than the Census. The NSSO includes persons with paralysis, amputation, deformity, dysfunction of joints and dwarfism as having locomotor disability. Persons with dwarfism or deformity are considered disabled even if they are not limited in the movement of their body or limbs. While in the Census, locomotor disability covers the absence of all toes, all fingers, deformity, and the inability to move without aid, the inability to lift and carry any small article as locomotor disability.

The estimates of mental disability proportion of disabled population are relatively close between the Census-2001 and the NSSO-2002 data. The proportion was (10.33 percent) as reported by the NSSO-2002 and (11.34 percent) reported by the Census 2001 data. The result is surprising, given the variations in the definitions taken for enumeration by the NSSO and the Census Operations. However in both sources, comprehension appropriate to age is used to capture persons with mental retardation. However, there are fundamental differences in the way mental illness is defined. The Census refers to persons who are "insane", while the NSSO identifies persons who exhibit behaviors like talking to self, laughing/crying, staring, violence, fear and suspicion without reason.

The definition of mental disability is also based on a general daily living limitation in the Census while it refers to several specific functional and activity of daily living limitations in the NSSO ["activities of communication (speech), self-care (cleaning of teeth, wearing clothes, taking bath, taking food, personal hygiene, etc.), home living (doing some household chores) and social skills"].

In the light of above discussion it is important to understand the global perspectives of defining disability in order to gather broader understanding of defining disability in India.

Defining Disability

Defining disability is difficult to accommodate the expectations of all disabled groups. There are hundreds of different disabilities and there are, as many causes for these disabilities. Some people are born with disabilities; others become disabled later on in their lives. Some disabilities exhibit themselves only periodically like fits and seizures; others are constant conditions and are life-long.[1] The severity of some stays the same, while others get progressively worse like muscular dystrophy and cystic fibrosis. Some are hidden and not obvious like epilepsy or haemophilia (impairment of blood clotting mechanism). Some disabilities can be controlled and cured while others still baffle the experts. Thus, finding a consensus on the different and frequently varying definitions of disabilities, whether sophisticated or practical, has never been easy. Some include total or partial impairment of senses and physical and intellectual capacities while defining disability. Others refer to a handicap or deviation of a social nature, injury or illness or incapacities to accomplish physiological functions or to obtain or keep employment.[2] These definitions also reflect the consequences for the individual – cultural, social, economic and environmental – that stem from the disability.

Helander[3]: Helander gave the simplest and may be the initial definition of a disabled person. "A person who in his/her society is regarded as disabled, because of a difference in appearances and/or behaviour." In most instances, a disabled person has functional limitations and/or activity restrictions. A 'functional limitation' disability may be defined as 'specific reductions in bodily functions that are described at the level of the person'. While 'Activity restriction' disability, may be defined as 'specific reductions in daily activities that are described at the level of the person'.

American Disability Act, 1990 (ADA)[4]

ADA defines individuals with physical or mental impairment. Persons having substantial limit of at least one major life activity or history of such impairment, and people who are regarded by others or perceived as having such impairment are defined as disabled. This definition protects people with epilepsy, diabetes, mental health conditions, amputees, and others who are able to mitigate the effects of their impairments but nonetheless encounter discrimination in the workplace and other settings because of fears, myths and stereotypes of individual employers and other covered entities. ADA has categorised disability in terms of physical and mental disability groups[5]:

> **Physical disability**: It includes . . . "Having any physiological disease, disorder, condition, cosmetic disfigurement, or anatomical loss that . . . affects one or more of the following body systems like: neurological, immunological, musculo-skeletal, special sense organs, respiratory, including speech organs, cardiovascular, reproductive, digestive, genitourinary, hemic and lymphatic, skin, and endocrine [and] limits a major life activity."

> **Mental disability**: It includes . . . "Having any mental or psychological disorder or condition, such as mental retardation, organic brain syndrome, emotional or mental illness, or specific learning disabilities, that limits a major life activity . . .".

Australia Disability Discrimination Act, 1972

Disability in relation to a person, means:[6]

(a) Total or partial loss of the person's bodily or mental functions; or
(b) Total or partial loss of a part of the body; or
(c) The presence in the body of organisms capable of causing disease or illness; or
(d) The presence in the body of organisms causing disease or illness; or
(e) The malfunction, malformation or disfigurement of a part of the person's body; or
(f) A disorder or malfunction that results in the person learning differently from a person without the disorder or malfunction; or
(g) A disorder, illness or disease that affects a person's thought processes, perception of reality, emotions or judgment or that results in disturbed behaviour and includes a disability that:

   (i) Presently exists; or
   (ii) Previously existed but no longer exists; or
   (iii) May exist in the future; or
   (iv) Is imputed to a person.

British Disability Discrimination Act, 1995

Disability is a physical or mental impairment, which has a substantial and long-term adverse effect on his ability to carry out normal day-to-day activities. In order to apply durability test, the British Act uses three different terms: loss of faculty, disability and disablement. These are meant to be separate concepts.

Loss of Faculty

Loss of faculty is any pathological condition or any loss or reduction of normal physical or mental functions of an organ or part of the body. A loss of faculty in itself may not be a disability but is an actual cause of one or more disabilities, e.g., the loss of one kidney.

Disability

A 'disability' means an inability to perform a normal bodily or mental process. It could either be complete inability to do something (such as walking) or it can be partial inability to do something (such as one can lift weights but not heavy ones).

Disablement

It is the sum total of all the separate disabilities an individual may suffer from. It means an overall inability to perform the normal activities of life and the loss of health, strength and power to enjoy a normal life.[7] While assessing an individual his/her physical and mental condition, inconvenience, genuine embarrassment or anxieties are taken into account.

India: Persons with Disabilities Act, 1995 (PWD-Equal opportunities, Protection of Rights and Full Participation)

Disability is defined a person suffering from not less than forty per cent of any disability as certified by a medical authority. The disabilities identified are; blindness, low vision, cerebral palsy, leprosy, leprosy cured, hearing impairment, locomotor disability, mental illness and mental retardation as well as multiple disabilities.

The National Sample Survey Organization (NSSO), India

The NSSO that conducted survey of persons with disabilities in 1981, 1991 and 2002 in India, considered disability as "Any restriction or lack of abilities to perform an activity in the manner or within the range considered normal for human being". It excludes illness/injury of recent origin (morbidity) resulting into temporary loss of ability to see, hears, speak or move.

International Labour Organization (ILO)

The ILO in its Vocational Rehabilitation and Employment (Disabled Persons) Convention defines a disabled person as an individual whose prospects of securing, retaining and advancing a suitable employment are substantially reduced as a result of duly recognised physical or mental impairment. The Declaration on the Rights of Disabled Persons, the term "Disabled Person" means, "Any person unable to ensure by himself or herself, wholly or partly, the necessities of a normal individual and/or social life as a result of deficiency, either congenital or not, in his or her physical or mental capabilities."[8]

United Nations: Standard rules on the Equalisation of Opportunities for Persons with Disabilities, 1994[9]

'Disability' summarises a great number of different functional limitations occurring in any population in any country of the world. People may be disabled by physical, intellectual or sensory impairment, medical conditions or mental illness. The term 'handicap' means the loss or limitation of opportunities to take part in the life of the community on an equal level with others. It describes the encounter between the persons with a disability and the environment. The purpose of this term is to emphasize the focus on the shortcomings in the environment and in many organised activities in society, e.g., information, communication and education, which prevent persons with disabilities from participating on equal terms.

World Health Organization: International Classification of Impairments, Disabilities and Handicaps (ICIDH) in 1980[10]

The ICIDH provides a conceptual framework for disability with three parts:

> Impairment is "any loss or abnormality of psychological, physiological, or anatomical structure or function". Impairments are disturbances at the level of the organ, which includes defects in or loss of a limb, organ or other body structure, as well as defects in or loss of a mental function. Examples of impairments include blindness, deafness, loss of sight in an eye, paralysis of a limb, amputation of a limb; mental retardation, partial sight, loss of speech, mutism, cerebral palsy and learning difficulties.
>
> **Disability** is a "restriction or lack (resulting from an impairment) of ability to perform an activity in the manner or within the range considered normal for a human being". It describes a functional limitation or activity restriction caused by impairment. Disabilities

are descriptions of disturbances in function at the level of the person. Examples of disabilities include difficulty in seeing, speaking or hearing; learning, difficulty in moving or climbing stairs; difficulty in grasping, reaching, bathing, eating, and toileting etc.

Handicap is a "disadvantage for a given individual, resulting from an impairment or disability, that limits or prevents the fulfillment of a role that is normal (depending on age, sex and social and cultural factors) for that individual". The term is also a classification of "circumstances in which disabled people are likely to find themselves". Handicap describes the social and economic roles of impaired or disabled persons that place them at a disadvantage compared to other persons. These disadvantages are brought about through the interaction of the person with specific environments and cultures. Examples of handicaps include being bedridden or confined to home; being unable to use public transport; being socially isolated, being forced to remain illiterate.

World Health Organization: International Classification of Impairments, Disabilities and Handicaps (ICIDH) in 2001

The document, referred to as the ICIDH-2, is officially titled the "International Classification of Functioning and Disability," or ICF.[11] Under this new system, the three concepts of impairment, disability and handicap have been replaced by two concepts –

- "Body functions and structures" (replacing "impairment"); and
- "Activities and participation" (replacing "handicap") – which are thoughts to extend the prior categories to permit the description of positive as well as negative experiences. The prior concept of "disability," or "functional" abilities or inabilities, is now conceived of as an umbrella concept applicable to either the body perspective, or to the individual and society perspective. The new system explicitly contemplates an assessment of "environmental factors,"

including the physical environment, the social environment and the impact of attitudes, and of "personal factors", which correspond to the personality and characteristic attributes of an individual.[12]

Disability Types

Disabled people do not form a homogenous group. They may be the physically disabled, mentally retarded, the visually, hearing and speech impaired, those with restricted mobility or with so-called "medical disabilities" and learning disabilities. They can broadly be classified as Physical and Communication, Mental, Learning and Medical disabilities.[13]

I. Physical and Communication Disabilities

Physical and Communication disabilities involve either loss of vision, physical movement, communication skills or a weakness or change in normal motor control. Some physical disabilities are present at birth (congenital) or are acquired due to illness, accident, or unknown causes. Loss of vision leads to complete blindness or low vision, loss of movement is often caused by spinal cord injury (damage to the nervous system) or by physical trauma such as severe fracture, burns or the amputation of a limb. One of the most common physical disabilities in young people is, cerebral palsy (CP). It produces disturbances of voluntary motor control ranging from clumsy and awkward movements to little or no coordinated movement. Individuals with CP can have related speech problems, as well as impaired hearing or vision. Other conditions such as muscular dystrophy, multiple sclerosis and amyotrophic lateral sclerosis, produce similar types of changes in physical functioning.

Visual impairment

Blindness: 'Blindness' refers to a condition where a person suffers from any of the following conditions, namely -total absence of sight; or visual acuity not exceeding 6/60 or 20/200 (snellen) in the better eye with correcting lenses; or limitation of the field of vision subtending an angle of 20 degrees or worse.

Person with low vision—A person with impairment of visual functioning even after treatment or standard refractive correction but who uses or is potentially capable of using vision for the planning or execution of a task with appropriate assistive device.

Hearing Impairment

Whose sense of hearing is non-functional for ordinary purposes in life? They do not hear/understand sound at all, even with amplified speech. The cases included in this category will be those having hearing loss of more than 60 decibels in the better ear (profound impairment) in the conversational range of frequency or total loss of hearing in both ears.

Locomotor Impairment

Locomotor impairment is disability of the bones, joint or muscles leading to substantial restriction of the movement of the limbs or a usual form of cerebral palsy and autism. Some common conditions giving raise to locomotor disability could be poliomyelitis, cerebral palsy, autism, amputation, injuries of spine, head, soft tissues, fractures, muscular dystrophies etc.

- **Orthopedic disability**: A persons inability to execute distinctive activities associated with moving both himself and objects, from place to place, and such inability resulting from affliction of either bones, joints, muscles or nerves. It could be poliomyelitis, amputation, injuries of spine, head, soft tissues, fractures, muscular dystrophies etc.
- **Cerebral Palsy:** A condition of Motor dysfunction of a person resulting from brain insult or injuries occurring in the pre-natal, peri- natal or infant period of development that affect movement control. The injury may be a brain infection (bacterial meningitis, viral encephalitis) or head injury before birth or following an accident.
- **Erb's Palsy, Brachial Plexus Palsy, or Shoulder Dystocia:** A condition when excessive lateral traction is applied to the fetal neck region during delivery. This can cause the Childs nerves to be torn, resulting in a limp arm. Tearing of these nerves can cause permanent paralysis of the arm.

- **Autism:** Autism is a complex developmental disability that typically appears during the first three years of life. It is the result of a neurological disorder that affects the functioning of the brain. It is a developmental disability typically affecting the processing, integrating, and organizing of information that significantly impacts communication, social interaction, functional skills, and educational performance.

Leprosy or 'Leprosy cured person' means any person who has been cured of leprosy but is suffering from –

- Loss of sensation in hands or feet as well as loss of sensation and paresis in the eye and eye-lid but with no manifest deformity;
- Manifest deformity and paresis but having sufficient mobility in their hands and feet to enable them to engage in normal economic activity;
- Extreme physical deformity as well as advanced age that prevent him from undertaking any gainful occupation, and the expression 'leprosy cured' shall be construed accordingly.

II. Mental, Psychological Illness and Mental Retardation

(a) **Mental, Psychological Illnesses:** These encompass Schizophrenia, anxiety disorders and depressive disorders. Schizophrenia is a highly complex disorder, which is caused due to a series of chemical changes in the brain. It usually occurs between the age groups of 15-25 years and is characterized by fragmented thoughts followed by an inability to process information. The condition affects the individual's family, professional and social life making him incapable of functioning normally. Surprisingly their intelligence is not affected and many of them are capable of leading partially normal life if they follow their regular pattern of medication and rehabilitation programmes such as those offered by half-way-homes.

(b) **Mental Retardation:** The definition includes 'any person who is unable to ensure himself/herself, wholly or partly, the necessities of a normal individual or social life including work, as a result of deficiency in his/her physical or mental capability'. A condition characterized by abnormal brain development in the womb not corresponding with normal physical growth. Their learning ability, reasoning power and judgment all develop at a slower pace. Accidents, poisoning, or illness after birth can be a cause for mental retardation. Many of the mentally retarded people are able to participate in activities with non-disabled people given an appropriate adaptation and support. Others may require a long-term structured programme. With adequate training and education such persons can be more self-reliant citizens. They can be found holding non-skilled or semi skilled jobs and can be made to effectively integrated into the social structure. Mental retardation is divisible into the following four categories.

1. Mild retardation IQ – 50-70
2. Moderate retardation IQ – 35-49
3. Severe retardation IQ – 20-34
4. Profound retardation IQ under 20

III. Learning Disabilities

It is a disorder, which affects the basic psychological processes of understanding or using written or spoken language. This disorder affects development of language, speech, reading and associated communication skills needed for social interaction. These children have deviant activity level, average or above average intelligence with perceptual disorders, problems in reading, writing, spelling and arithmetic, delayed or slow development of speech articulation, short attention span, frequent changes in mood, low self esteem, low or below average social competence, impulsive, problems in motor activities and spatial organization, poor temporal concepts, passive, lacking strategies for tackling academic problems, having inadequate grasp of what strategies are available for problem solving and do not believe in their abilities.

Conditions such as brain injury, minimal brain dysfunction, dyslexia, and developmental aphasia are examples of learning disabilities.

- **Dyslexia:** Affect persons ability to acquire, process, and/or use either, spoken, read, written or nonverbal information (organization/planning, functional literacy skills, memory, reasoning, problem solving, perceptual skills) or in other words in short- difficulty with language in its various uses (not always reading).

- **Dysgraphia:** Difficulty with the act of writing both in the technical as well as the expressive sense. There may also be difficulty with spelling.
- **Dyscalculia:** Difficulty with calculations.
- **Attention Deficit and Hyperactivity Disorder (ADHD).**

IV. Multiple Disabilities

A combination of two or more disabilities as defined in clause (i) of section 2 of the Person with disabilities (Equal Opportunities, Protection of Rights and Full Participation) Act, 1995 namely Blindness/low vision Speech and Hearing impairment Locomotor disability including leprosy cured Mental retardation and Mental illness.

V. Medical Disabilities

A medical disability can be defined as a condition that requires intervention such as medical treatment, prescription drugs, and/or accommodation to help a person participate in life's activities. Medical disabilities may be acute or chronic, visible or invisible, and the type of support needed is diverse. The chronic health problems include fibromyalgia, chronic fatigue syndrome, arthritis, kidney disease, allergies, cardiovascular problems, cancer, diabetes, and HIV infections, as well as respiratory and gastro-intestinal disorders. Recognizing medical conditions may be difficult because many are 'hidden'. The primary diagnosis may be accompanied by secondary impairments in mobility, vision, hearing, speech, or coordination depending on the nature and/or progression of the condition. Medical disabilities can be classified into:

Autoimmune Illness: It includes fibromyalgia, chronic fatigue syndrome, rheumatoid arthritis, asthma and lupus. A lowered immunity can result in frequent illnesses. Patients can experience flare-ups, side effects of medication, or hospitalisation.

Blood serum disorders: It include haemophilia, thalassemia, sickle cell anaemia, HIV/AIDS, and other disorders. Blood serum disorders can be characterized by severe crisis periods with extreme pain and other complications, which may necessitate hospitalisation.

Epilepsy: It is a disorder of the central nervous system, which results in a seizure. For many adults, epileptic seizures are largely controlled by anti-convulsion medication. There are four major kinds of seizures, distinguished by the degree of convulsion and the extent to which the person is conscious. Grand mal epilepsy involves sudden and violent convulsions and loss of consciousness, whereas Petit mal epilepsy is milder and involves little or no loss of consciousness. The person may stop what he/she is doing and stare momentarily.

Cancers: It can occur in almost any organ system of the body, the systems and particular disabling effects will vary greatly from one person to another. People may experience visual problems, lack of balance and coordination, joint pain, backaches, headaches, abdominal pain, drowsiness, lethargy, difficulty in breathing and swallowing, weakness, bleeding, or anaemia. The primary treatments for cancer can cause additional effects such as violent nausea, drowsiness, and fatigue. Medical treatment can result in amputation, paralysis, sensory deficits, and language and memory problems.

Cystic Fibrosis (CF): It is a disease affecting the cells lining the pancreas, small intestines, sweat glands, and lungs. CF's respiratory symptoms are chronic and eventually lead to fatal lung infections.

Muscular Dystrophy: It refers to a group of hereditary, progressive disorders that most often occur with young people, producing degeneration of voluntary muscles of the trunk and extremities. Atrophying of muscles results in chronic weakness and fatigue and may cause respiratory or cardiac problems. Walking, if possible, is slow.

Multiple Sclerosis: is a progressive disease of the central nervous system, characterized by a decline of muscle control. Symptoms range from mild to severe and may include blurred vision, legal blindness, tremors, weakness or numbness in limbs, unsteady gait, paralysis, slurred speech, mood swings, or attention deficits. Periodic remissions are common and may last from a few days to several months as the disease continues to progress.

Drug and Alcohol Abuse: Persons who are in treatment programs experience psychological problems such as depression, anxiety, or low self-esteem, as well as cognitive deficits such as impaired concentration or short-term memory.

Concluding Remarks and Recommendations

In the light of above stated discussion it is important to cover all major types of disability types in our Census and other national data sources of enumeration, so as to prepare realistic policy programmes and effectively address the issues of disabled.

As noted above, three disability type definitions (hearing, speech and locomotor) are more inclusive in the NSSO than in the Census Operations. The reverse is true for visual disability where the Census definition is wider than that in the NSSO. The vast differences in prevalence estimates between the Census and the NSSO, illustrate how essential it is to document the disability definition used, sources and caveats and to exercise great caution while comparing prevalence estimates or using statistics related to disability.

In the Census, the definitions of disability types can be improved as follows:

(i) There are inconsistencies across disability types as to whether the functional limitation applies to a situation where an assistive device is used. For locomotor disability, it refers to a person's limitation without using aid while for hearing; it refers to a limitation experienced despite the use of hearing aid. Such inconsistencies certainly make it difficult for field staff to collect the data and for researchers to interpret the results.

(ii) In addition, in the Census, the term 'insane' is used to define mental illness: this term is subjective and using it to classify persons seems inadequate.

(iii) Finally, the definition of visual disability needs to be narrowed down so that persons who have mild visual limitations and have not been tested for vision acuity are not counted as disabled.

As for the NSSO, the definitions of disability and disability types and the scope of disability data collection should be revised as follows:

(i) The current definitions of disability and disability types are a mix of activity limitation (general definition, visual and mental disability), functional limitations (e.g., speech) and impairments (in locomotor disability, dwarfs and persons with stiff neck of permanent nature who generally do not have difficulty in the normal movement of body and limbs will also be treated as disabled). As a result, it is unsure what exactly the NSSO based prevalence estimate encompasses. There should be separate questions getting at impairments, functional and activity limitations.

(ii) There is scope for improving data collection on disability by including disability questions in non disability schedules in the NSSO. Fewer than a handful of disability questions would facilitate the comparison of the welfare of persons with and without disabilities. A disadvantage of the data from schedule 26 is that it only covers Persons with Disability (PWDs), and makes it therefore impossible to compare the welfare of persons with and without disabilities at a given point in time. For instance, in the rounds of the NSSO that collect employment data for large samples (e.g., 55th round), PWDs are not identified. As a result, some questions that are essential to understanding the standard of living of PWDs cannot be tackled with existing data. Is there discrimination in access to employment against PWDs? Is there underemployment among PWDs? Adding disability questions to selected rounds of the NSSO could go a long way in giving researchers the data needed to try and answer these questions.

REFERENCES

1. Brown, Scott Campbell (2001). "Methodological paradigms that shape disability research," chap. 5 in Gary L. Albrecht, Katherine D. Seelman and Michael Bury (eds.) *Handbook of Disability Studies* (Thousand Oaks, Sage Publications, 2001), p. 164.

2. Pechansky, R. and Thomas, C. (1981). "The Concept of Access: Definition and Relation to Customer Satisfaction." *Medical Care*, vol. 19, no. 2, p. 128.
3. Helander, Einar. *Prejudice and Dignity: An Introduction to Community Based Rehabilitation*. UNDP, New York.
4. National Council of Disability, Americans With Disability Act, 1990. Policy Brief Series, February, 2003.
5. Disability Act Policy Brief Series: Righting the ADA, Defining 'Disability' in a Civil Rights Context: The Courts' Focus on Extent of Limitations as Opposed to Fair Treatment and Equal Opportunity.
6. Disability Discrimination Act, 1992. Australian Government.
7. Whiteneck, Gale G., Patrick Fougeyrollas and Kenneth A. Gerhart (1997). "Elaborating the model of disablement," in Marcus J. Fuher (ed.) Assessing medical rehabilitation practices: the promise of outcomes research (Baltimore, Paul H. Brookes Publishing) pp. 99-100.
8. Economic and Social Council document E/2000/L.9 <http://www.un.org/documents/ecosoc/docs/2000/e2000-l9.pdf>.
9. The Standard Rules on the Equalisation of Opportunities for Persons with Disabilities. 1994. United Nations.
10. International Classification of Impairments, Disabilities and Handicaps (ICIDH), World Health Organization, Geneva, 1980, p.180.
11. See ICIDH-2: International Classification of Functioning and Disability, available at http://www.ncd.gov/newsroom/publications/www.deakin.edu.au/tedca/ncet/information/resources/ididh.html
12. Ibid.
13. Refer details in brochure of, Chaffey College - 5885 Haven Avenue - Rancho Cucomonga, California 91737.

3

Strategies for Including the Excluded: The Differently Abled

Asha J.V.

There is a general perception that students with certain disabilities can only thrive under special circumstances and hence are best left to special schools/institutions. But, in fact, by putting them in a certain special school/institution, we are killing their confidence and their belief that they can live and be successful in any environment. These children are not disabled in any way. They are differently-abled and have their own way of coming up in life. A little bit of confidence from our side will push their confidence levels and make them aim for higher goals. It is estimated that more than 500 million people in the world are disabled as a consequence of mental, physical or sensory impairment and of this 80 million belong to India. At every minute a few are added to this multi category group as victims of war, violence, terrorism, accidents, malnutrition, illiteracy and inadequate health practices (Biswas, 2004).

Worldwide, there has been a conscious shift away from special schooling to mainstream. On the international platform there has been a number of encouraging pronouncements in recent years for combating the discriminatory attitude by creating welcoming communities, building an inclusive society and improving the efficiency by enhancing cost effectiveness of the entire educational system. The UN Convention (1981) on the Right of the child, initiatives of UNESCO and World Bank (1994), WHO (1997) etc. took bold steps on the equalization of opportunities for persons with disabilities.

Laws and Policies Regarding Inclusion

Though service to disabled children in India is more than 100 years old, the coverage of these children in the formal school system is not even 5 per cent. The education of children with disability has been discussed as part of the National Policy on Education (NPE, 1986) and its Programme of Action (POA, 1992). Still, a large number of students hesitate to join the University due to inadequate facilities to participate on an equal basis with other members of the University in the teaching and learning process. However, the last decade witnessed the passing and implementation of three major legislations on disability both at central and state levels; viz., Rehabilitation Council of India (RCI) Act, 1992, Persons with Disability Act, 1995 and National Trust Act, 1999. The Ministry of of Human Resource Development (MHRD) is currently in the process of developing a comprehensive Action Plan on inclusive education for children and youth with disabilities. A statement spelling out the areas of action has made in the Rajya Sabha by Sri Arjun Singh, the Minister, HRD on 21st March, 2005. The different sectors covered by the plan are: (1) Early Childhood Care, (2) Elementary Education, (3) Secondary Education, (4) Higher and Technical Education, (5) Vocational Education. Thus under the Integrated Education for Disabled Children Scheme of the MHRD, over 1.24 lakh children with disabilities have been integrated over 20000 main stream schools. At the Elementary level, under SSA programme, over 14 lakh children with disabilities have been enrolled. The report of manpower development published by the Rehabilitation Council of India (RCI) reveals that Bachelor's and Master's level teacher preparation programmes are needed for preparing teachers to help disabled children realise the objective 'education for all'. The University Grants Commission (UGC) had already announced that they would support selected university departments and colleges of education in the country to offer special education, with financial assistance available under the programme of Integrated Education for Disabled Children by the Ministry of Human Resource Development, Government of India, or within the available resources of the UGC. The UGC had started the scheme of assistance to universities/colleges to facilitate Teacher Preparation in Special Education (TEPSE) and Higher Education for Persons with Special Needs (Differently-abled Persons) (HEPSN) during the Ninth Five-Year Plan itself, keeping in view the need to provide special education programmes as well as infrastructure to differently-abled persons. The infrastructure needs to be designed in a manner to enable them to easily access classrooms, laboratories, toilets, etc. In addition, innovations in technology made available a variety of assistive tools designed to help the differently-abled. However, according to NSSO (2002) figures of the literate disabled population, only 9 percent completed secondary level and above education.

Integrated education is the term which refers to integration of special needs students in general education where they receive education at par with others whereas inclusive education is a developmental approach seeking to address the learning needs of all children, youth and adults with specific focus on those who are vulnerable to marginalization and exclusion. It is in fact a ray of hope that exerts a positive impact on the awareness of the community when there would be more interactions between the disabled individuals and non-disabled individuals, which contribute to both bonding and building the society. Thus inclusion becomes a moral issue, a goal, indeed a value we decide to pursue or reject on the basis of what we want our society to look like (Biswas, 2004). So inclusive education, as a concept or notion requires educational institutions to respond to the varying competencies of the student rather than students adapting to the institution and the curriculum practices. This in turn envisages a system which fulfils the goal of National Knowledge Commission (2007): 'expansion, excellence and inclusion'.

The Major Barriers

The process of exclusion and inclusion are inextricably linked.

An analysis of the system brings out that the pressure towards exclusion is very important to understand inclusion. It is because within the same system the same individuals may be encouraged or discouraged from participation. The real challenge of inclusive education is to meet the special needs of all individuals with and without disabilities. Thus it becomes clear that inclusion is not a soft process and that it requires commitment to overcome all types of barriers. The major barriers identified can be listed as: Systemic barriers, Pedagogic barriers and Psycho-social barriers.

Systemic barriers include: (a) lack of basic and appropriate support materials/supportive services, (b) lack of assistive devices, (c) lack of disabled friendly infrastructure, (d) lack of peripheral services.

The major *pedagogic barriers* are: (a) insufficient support from educators, (b) inappropriate and unfair evaluation, (c) rigid curricular frame work.

Psycho-social barriers can differ from society to society. Some of the barriers included in this category are: (a) attitudinal factors, (b) severe poverty, (c) late enrolment, (d) lack of early intervention programme, (e) gender issues in cultural groups and society, (f) lack of access to basic services.

Bold Steps

The University of Delhi and a few institutions in India have committed themselves to provide all possible facilities to the differently-abled irrespective of visual, hearing, orthopaedic, or other kinds of impairment. Their mission is to enable all differently-abled students and staff to participate fully in the academic, intellectual, social, and cultural life of the University and society (Draft Report, University of Delhi). This noble ideal has been envisaged by many universities of the developed nations. Human rights are essentially to secure freedom, in quest of 'well being and dignity of all people everywhere (HDR, 2000). The development experience of Kerala usually named the 'Kerala model' highlights the high level of social development and physical quality of life disproportionate to its low level of economic development. In the context of the paradigm shift in the concept and measures of development from economic development to human development, Kerala's development process got much significance in promoting human development. However, the efficiency of the State to provide equal educational opportunities to disabled/differently-abled persons in higher education institutions still remains an enigma. To identify the educational as well as infrastructural barriers that try to exclude the differently-abled persons is an area which demands imminent attention.

Tips to Tackle Differently-abled in Classroom

A discussion with experts in the field and review of literature (Pandey and Advani, 1995; Panda, 2000; Julka, 2005; Singal, 2005b) suggest the following practices to be effective ways to retain the differently abled in the classrooms:

- Include or allow the child to participate in school activities à academic activities, lunch time activities, recess games etc... if she/he can
- Provide least restrictive environment
- Requires new models of collaboration
- Develop Individual Education Plan (IEP)
- Teachers are responsible for instructional decisions
- Decide on developmentally appropriate content and process

Preparing Teachers for Diverse Learners: The Strategies

An unstructured, informal inquiry with the teacher educators pointed out that there should be provision in teacher preparation courses to initiate the prospective teachers in the areas of special education. They also suggested the following aspects to be taken up as strategies for preparing diverse learners in classrooms:

- Making more explicit institutional commitments in the areas of recruitment, admissions, curriculum infusion, conferences and forums, university and field enquiries (extension activities).
- More systematic and explicit attention to be given to issues such as equity, inclusion and social justice.
- Efforts to offer a more diversified curriculum and relevant pedagogy at the secondary level.

- Teacher recruitment is to be purely on the basis of merit.
- The transition from students of teaching to teachers of students is a difficult one.

ICT and Inclusion

In recent years there has been an unprecedented increase in the availability of information and communication technology (ICT) tools to support learners with additional needs. Students with special needs are now having a greater impact on the general education system and the percentage of students with disabilities served in schools classes with their non disabled peers has gradually increased. As the size and numbers of students classified as special needs students increase, the scope of assistive technology in schools is also growing in importance. The use of technology may allow students to compensate for their disability or circumvent it entirely.

Assistive Tools

The term "assistive tools" means any item, piece of equipment, or product system, whether acquired commercially off the shelf, modified, or customized that is used to increase, maintain, or improve functional capabilities of a child with a disability. They are software and hardware products used by the differently-abled to accomplish their task easily and to lead an independent life. In the early days this included huge, bulky and cumbersome hardware which either stood alone, or was attached to a computer. Now this has changed to a more integrated system. According to Lewis (1998), assistive technology serves two major purposes: to augment an individual's strengths, thereby counterbalancing the effects of the disability, and to provide an alternative mode of performing a task. Thus, the use of technology allows students to compensate for their disability or circumvent it entirely.

Assistive technology is often discussed by technology levels as being high-, middle-, or low-tech. A low-tech assistive technology option is usually easy to use, has low cost, and typically does not require a power source. Mid-tech assistive devices are also easy to operate but typically require a power source. The high-tech device is usually complex and programmable, and usually includes items that require computers, electronics or microchips to perform a function. The following are the commonly used assistive tools:

Braille and Refreshable Braille—This is an electro-mechanical device for displaying Braille characters, usually by means of raising dots through holes in a flat surface.

Alternative Keyboards—These have been designed for people who have difficulty in using their hands or who use foot.

Screen Magnifiers

Here we are talking about software that interfaces with a computer's graphical output to present enlarged screen content.

Screen Readers—This is a software application that attempts to identify and interpret what is being displayed on the screen. E.g., JAWS, SAFA, and ORCA.

Speech Recognition—It converts spoken words to machine-readable input and is especially useful for people having difficulty in using their hands.

Speech Synthesizers—It involves the artificial production of human-like speech. E.g. Festival and *e*Speak.

Voice Browsers—A Web browser that presents an interactive voice user interface to the user is known as a Voice Browser.

There is no dearth of expensive assistive technological products in the market. It is not mere the lack of awareness that deters people from using it, but they are very costly and unaffordable by Indian standards. Most disabled people in India are simply not affluent enough to afford it and this prevents many people with disabilities from acquiring the assistive devices which would enable them to be mobile and participate in programmes for their economic and social well-being. This calls for the need for indigenous development of low cost assistive devices.

The potential for assistive technology in higher education classrooms for students with disabilities is great. Its benefits include enhancing academic achievement in written expression, reading, mathematics, and spelling; improving organization and fostering social acceptance. They enable many learners with access- difficulties to overcome barriers. Physical, sensory and learning difficulties can be supported by their use. Assistive tools have the capacity to increase student independence and participation in classroom activities and simultaneously advancing academic standing for students with special needs, providing them the ability to have equal access to their learning environment *(Asha, 2009)*.

The Kerala Context

There are initiatives in Kerala for bridging the divide between the disabled and the "abled' inside integrated classrooms. The Social Welfare Department is running special educational institutions catering to the need of these students. The National Institute of Speech and Hearing, Akulam is one such institute and they are offering four different courses for this special category students; three at under graduate level and one at post graduate level. Even though we acclaim the issues of access, equity, accountability and quality as the four guiding principles, while planning for higher education development in the twenty-first century, it is a bare fact that the access factor and equity factor of the deprived sections in general and that of the differently-abled in particular are met with only when the other two factors viz., accountability and quality are maintained. The institutions are to be made accountable for providing necessary infrastructural facilities to these categories of students. For this, brisk paced measures to make the institutions disabled-friendly are required along with equipping teachers to handle heterogeneous classrooms. Some suggestions derived from the discussion with teacher educators include:

- The curriculum should be made more flexible with inbuilt provisions for adapting instruction as per the requirement of the learner and making viable norms of evaluation according to the level of the learner and the differing ability displayed.
- The higher education scenario, especially teacher preparation courses are to take bold steps to bring in the change. Along with this, awareness campaigns also need to be organized in order to make the public also involved in the process of inclusion.

- For realizing the concept of inclusive society that can provide the foundations for a knowledge society, an exhaustive and systematic overhaul in education, especially in higher education is imperative.
- Education institutions also have to make suitable infra-structural facilities or to avoid systemic barriers to equip the differently-abled non-parasitic individuals and help them to bloom to the fullest possible ways of self reliance and confidence.

REFERENCES

Asha, J.V. (2009) *Equipping Strategies for the Differently-abled*, key note address in National Seminar on "*Student Progression: An Integrated Guidance and Counselling Perspective*", www. fmtcpallimukku.org.

Julka, A. (2005) *Educational Provisions and Practices for Learners with Disabilities in India*, paper presented at the Inclusive and Supportive Education Congress 2005, University of Strathclyde, Glasgow accessed through google disability pdf.

Mani, M.N.G. (2002). Inclusive Education. Paper presented at the Inclusion International Congress 2002, Melbourne, Australia.

NCERT, (1998). Sixth Survey in Education. New Delhi.

Panda, P. (2005) *Responsiveness of Pre-service Teacher Education Programme Towards Inclusive Education in India: Appraisal of Curriculum Dimensions and Practices*, ational Council of Educational Research and Training paper presented at the Inclusive and Supportive Education Congress 2005, University of Strathclyde, Glasgow.

Rehabilitation Council of India (1996). 9th Annual Report (1995-96). New Delhi, RCI.

Singal, N. (2005b) *Mapping the field of inclusive education: A review of the Indian literature*, International Journal of Inclusive Education, 9 (4), October-December 2005, pp. 331-350.

Sreerekha, R. (2009) *ICT Alternatives To Inclusion—A Case Study in Kerala Perspective*; Paper Presented at International Conference On '*Education, Research And Innovations For Inclusive Societies*', March 19-21, Kuppam.

The Salamanca Statement and Framework for Action on Special Needs Education (1994). Presentation at the World Conference on Special Needs Education: Access and Quality at Salamanca, 1994.

Web References

http://www.braillewithoutborders.org
http://computing.in.msn.com
http://www.disabilityindia.com/html/assistivetechnology.html
http://insight.kerala.gov.in
http://jakemp.nic.in/schemes/scheme7.htm
www.rehabcouncil.nic.in
http://socialjustice.ekduniya.net

4

Disability and Skill Development in India

Rakesh Raman Jha

Disability has deeper understanding of human right dimension and often associated with social exclusion, increased exposure and vulnerability to poverty.[1] Thus disability is the outcome of complex interactions between the functional limitations arising from a person's physical, intellectual, or mental condition and social and physical environment. It has multi dimension and thus have a broader perspective of national health and medical problem.

Peggy Quinn in his book *Understanding Disability: a lifespan approach*[2] argues that social workers and other health and mental health professionals are now encountering people with a wide range of disabilities at various stages of their lives. It is important to be prepared. Understanding disability details expected developmental stages for those without disabilities as well as the impact of disability at each of these periods. This is a much needed reference for working with a person with a disability, or with a family member or other interested party. Beginning with infancy and the diagnosis of congenital or early onset disabilities, the book identifies traditional developmental life stages and then provides specific information for four different disabilities: Down syndrome, visual impairment, cerebral palsy, and spina bifida. In addition, spinal cord injury is added at the young adult stage of some adapted expectations. In keeping with a social work emphasis on strengths, he argues that disability is social, rather than medical.

Maureen Lovett[3] explains that the constructs of accuracy and speed were adopted as performance criteria. Accuracy-disabled subjects had failed to achieve reliable age-appropriate word recognition skills. Rate-disabled readers were age-appropriate in word recognition accuracy but deficient in reading speed. These disabled readers were compared to fluent normal children selected to be reading at the same level of accuracy as the rate-disabled subjects but at a significantly faster rate. All aspects of the accuracy-disabled subjects' reading systems proved deficient, and these children were less able to learn new sound-symbol associations in a task simulating initial reading acquisition. The rate-disabled subjects exhibited a basic deficit in word recognition speed, compromised accuracy when reading in context, and compromised spelling when competing visual patterns were available. Multidimensional oral language impairment was found to accompany the accuracy disability, while the rate disability appeared restricted to language in its visible form and the naming of visual representations. Visual naming speed impairment was associated with both profiles of deficient reading skill.

The WHO argues that 50 per cent of disabilities are preventable and directly linked to poverty. Worldwide there are 1.5 million blind children exits mainly in Africa and Asia. In developing countries, up to 70 per cent of blindness in children is either preventable or treatable. The WHO also estimates that 50 per cent of disabling hearing impairment is also preventable.[4]

There is an important and fundamental difference between disability and other forms of disadvantage. People with disabilities can only organise themselves to claim their rights when their additional practical needs, such as for mobility aids, have been met. People with disabilities have a right to be included in all aspects of life.[5] In order to fight for the right to inclusion, people with disabilities need to live in an environment in which they are empowered.

People with disabilities face numerous barriers in realizing equal opportunities; environmental and access barriers, legal and institutional barriers, and attitudinal barriers which cause social exclusion. Social exclusion is often the hardest barrier to overcome, and is usually associated with feelings of shame, fear and rejection. An increasingly common criticism of traditional approaches to disability, particularly from people with disabilities themselves, is that their needs have been marginalized by being categorized as 'special' or 'different' from those of the population at large.[6] Conventional approaches have been criticised for being driven by a perception that people with disabilities need help to adapt to society's demands. This approach runs the risk of favouring technical or medical solutions that emphasize difference rather than promote inclusion.[7]

Health and fitness, as well as gender and age, affect the likelihood of people benefiting from development programmes in their communities. According to some sources, as many as one person in ten has a disability.[8] Three out of four are thought to live in developing countries. 'Disability limits access to education and employment, and leads to economic and social exclusion. Poor people with disabilities are caught in a vicious cycle of poverty and disability, each being a cause and a consequence of the other'.[9]

Therefore, the Constitution of India emphasizes the protection of the disabled person basic right. Article 41 of the constitution of India calls upon the governments at all levels to make effective provision for securing the right to work, to establish and to publish assistance in cases of unemployment.[10] Another relevant provision of the Constitution is entry 9 of state list relating to relief of the disabled and unemployment.[11] The parliament of India with this principles adopted "The Persons with Disability (Equal Opportunities, Protection of Rights and Full Participation) Act, 1995". The act is the main legal document for protection of the disabled person in the country. It defined that a person suffering from not less than forty percent of any disability as certified by a medical authority is identified as disabled person. In addition, the definition of disability is divided into seven groups, blindness, low vision, leprosy cured, hearing impairment, locomotor disability, mental retardation and mental illness.[12]

The government of India in the general census started registering the total disabled person in the country. The 2001 census estimated that India has total 21,906,769 disabled people. Among them 16,388,382 is living in rural areas and 5,518,387 lives in urban areas. The total number of male disabled (12,605,635) is higher than the female disabled (9,301,134) in the country.[13] The census of 1991 were approximately calculated 16 million people with visual impairment, hearing impairment and locomotor disabilities in India in that year, constituting about 1.9 per cent of the population.[14]

According to 58th Sample Survey conducted by NSSO in 2002, indicate that there are about 18.04 million persons with various types of disabilities in the country. Their disabilities restrict the opportunity for their economic and social growth. In addition, about 3 per cent of the children below 14 years of age suffer from delayed development and found that 29 out of 1,000 children in the urban areas (2.9 per cent) and 30 out of 1,000 children (3 per cent) in the rural areas had developmental delays associated with mental disability. The estimated number of persons with disabilities working in 1991 constituted 4.52 million leaving 0.08 million (1.7 per cent) unemployed. Many of them are mentally retarded and cerebral palsied and require some aids/appliances to attain the capacity for self-care and independent living.[15]

The distribution of disabled people by employment status is given in Table 1.

Table 1. Employment Status of People with Disabilities at Work in 1991 (millions)

Status	Rural	Urban	Total
Self-Employment Agriculture	1.65	0.07	1.72
Self-Employment Non-Agriculture	0.52	0.37	0.89
Regular Employee	0.25	0.28	0.53
Casual Labour	1.18	0.20	1.38
Total	3.60	0.92	4.52

Source: ILO, March, 2003. *Employment of People with Disabilities: The Impact of Legislation (India Country Profile)*, ILO in Focus Programme on Skills, Knowledge and Employability, Development Cooperation Ireland.

Of the 16 million disabled people identified in 1991, as many as 11.4 million did not participate in the labour force. Table 2 indicates their activity status.

Table 2. Activity status of unemployed disabled people (millions) 1991

Status	Rural		Urban		Total	
	1991	2001	1991	2001	1991	2001
Attending education	1.37		0.64		2.01	
Attending domestic work	1.68		0.55		2.23	
Beggars	0.09		0.03		0.12	
Other	5.59		1.43		7.02	
Total	8.73		2.65		11.38	

Source: ILO, March, 2003. *Employment of People with Disabilities: The Impact of Legislation (India Country Profile)*, ILO in Focus Programme on Skills, Knowledge and Employability, Development Cooperation Ireland.

In the tenth plan period, during 2003-04 budgets, Central Government allocated Rs. 274 crore for the policy programmes of the disabled. It was 17 per cent of the total plan allocation of the MSJE. An expenditure of Rs. 248 crore was incurred during the period. It was 19.8 per cent of the total expenditure of the ministries for the disabled. During the period 130 districts are selected to provide comprehensive services for the disabled persons in the country. 107 district disability centers were set up during the period. The expert committee on social welfare has identified 120 jobs at the supervisory, executive and managerial levels and 945 jobs at the level of skilled/semi skilled suitable for person with disabilities, in the private sector.[16]

In the tenth plan approach paper, a general development plan for all of India, that inclusion of people with disabilities in all sphere of life including vocational training and employment has been incorporated. The central government formulated a national policy on disability as well as a national programme for action in consonance with the world programme for action adopted during the international decade of disabled persons during 1983–92. The following two main focus areas were adopted which are (i) Effective implementation of the Person with Disabilities Act, 1995 to ensure social justice to disabled with equitable terms and (ii) Strengthening and Consolidating of the outreach and extension programmes through National Programme for Rehabilitation of Persons with Disabilities.[17] A comprehensive law on the entitlement and programme for persons with disabilities in all areas including education, vocational training and employment, rehabilitation, accessibility, institutional care etc. has been included. Although there are no specific provision for disability in the existing labour codes or other legislation relating to education, vocational training and employment.[18]

Skill Training and Disability in India

For a normal person, training is required for development of skills to earn good livelihoods. But for a disabled person, there are two types of training required. First to learning method without specific organs and then there is another training needs for providing livelihoods.[19] Therefore, for a disabled person providing training is needed a highly specialised training facilities so one person could stand without specific organ.

The Government of India since eight five year plan has been focusing to provide specific assistance to the million of the dísabled persons in the country. There are six national institute working for the welfare and rehabilitation of persons with disability (PWDs). These institutes work in the fields of locomotors, visual, hearing and mental disability. There are two other organisation are working for PWDs.[20] These are 'National Handicapped Finance and Development Corporation (NHFDC) and Artificial Limbs Manufacturing Corporation of India Ltd. (ALIMCO)'. The basic objective of first one is to promote economic empowerment of PWDs through financing self employment ventures and assisting beneficiaries in he up gradation of technical and entrepreneurship skill for effective management of their self employment ventures.[21]

Under the Ministry of Social Justice and Empowerment (MSJE), National Trust was established for the welfare of persons with autism, cerebral palsy, mental Retardation and multiple Disabilities. The basic works of the trust is to provide opportunities to the disabled person to live to their live as independently and as possible within or close to their own communities. The trust works with organisation working for the disabled person to provide training facilities to empower them for decent livelihoods. The trust establishes 369 local level committees in 26 states and 4 UT.[22] There are 11 district rehabilitation centres through out India. This basic objective is to provide comprehensive rehabilitation services to PWDs in rural areas. It was established in 1993 and the objectives of the council are to regulate training policies and programme in the field of rehabilitation of PWDs and to regulate standard for PWDs in all training institutions uniformly through the country.[23]

Along with these, the MSJE have other national institutes. These are: (i) national institute for Orthopaedically Handicapped, (ii) National institute for the mentally handicapped, (iii) Ali Yavar Jung National institute for hearing Handicapped, (iv) national institute for the Visually Handicapped, (v) National institute of rehabilitation Training and Research, and (vi) Institute for the Physically Handicapped.[24] These institutes provide vocational training and employment to those disabled person who have specific disability. Even these institutes provide training to the professionals and grassroots workers to upgrade their knowledge and skills to give training to the disabled persons.

The other ministries in the government of India also have specific programme for the skill training facilities for the person with disabilities. These ministries are ministry of health and family welfare, Ministry of Urban affairs and Employment, Ministry of Rural Development and Employment, Ministry of Human Resource Development, Ministry of Labour, Ministry of Railways, Ministry of civil aviations, Department of Science and Rechnology, Department of woman and Child Development.

The main function of the Central Coordination Committee is to serve as the national focal point on disability matters and facilitate the continuous evolution of a comprehensive policy towards solving the problems faced by persons with disabilities.[25] The Committee reviews and coordinates the activities of all the Departments of Government and other Governmental and non-Governmental Organisations that deal with matters relating to persons with disabilities. It is also involved in the development of a national policy to address issues faced by persons with disabilities and as a necessary corollary advises the Central Government on the formulation of policies, programmes, legislation and projects with respect to disability. It has the authority to take up the cause of persons with disabilities with the concerned authorities and the international organisations with a view to provide for schemes and projects for the disabled in the national plans and other programmes and policies evolved by the international agencies.[26] In this respect it consults with donor agencies to review their funding policies from the perspective of their impact on persons with disabilities.

The Rehabilitation Council of India was set up as a registered society in 1986 under the aegis of the Ministry of Social Justice & Empowerment (then Ministry of Social Welfare) to standardize and maintain uniform standards of training of professionals. However, it was soon realised that the Society could not ensure proper standardization and acceptance of the standards by other Organizations. The Parliament enacted the Rehabilitation Council of India Act in 1992. The Rehabilitation Council of India became a Statutory Body on 22 June 1993.[27]

Along with the central and the state government various organisation for the protection of the disabled persons in the country, several NGO also play an important role in promoting employment opportunities with disabilities in India. Among the NGO, national centre for the promotion of employment of disabled people is the largest which advocate and promote equality for persons with disabilities in all spheres of life, through education, communication, appropriate training and barrier free environment for gainful employment. The other NGOs that specifically target the employment of people with disabilities include the 'association of people with disabilities'; 'action on disability and development'; and Narajeevana. The MSJE supports 644 institutions for running early intervention programmes, special education programmes, vocational training programmes under which 1600 people are covered. Among them 190 NGOs runs Vocational Training Programmes for PWDs from 1992-2000.[28] In response to the ILO Convention No. 159 concerning Vocational Rehabilitation and Employment of Disabled Persons (1983) policy on employment opportunities for people with disabilities is frequently supported by legislation and implementation strategies as essential tools to promote integration and social inclusion, Many countries throughout the world have, in recent years, adopted policies aiming to promote the rights of people with disabilities to full and equal participation in society.

The Director-General of Employment and Training under the Ministry of Labour have programme for Persons with disabilities to provide an appropriate job through country's employment exchange. Special Employment Exchanges is also running over three decades for their selective placement. These exchanges attempt to secure for the disabled the most satisfying form of employment suitable to their residual physical and mental potentialities. At present, 42 Special Exchanges are functioning. In addition to this, 41 Special Cells for disabled persons with a Special Placement Officer attached to the normal Employment Exchanges and funded by the Central Government have so far been set up by the Ministry of Social Justice and Empowerment.[29]

In addition to this, NGOs also run their placement services for specific category of disability. Under this scheme, Placement officers follow up with the training institutions for people with disabilities and also with the employers to identify vacancies. These Placement Officers also match the skills of disabled persons with the available job and try to secure actual placement.[30] The Ministry of Social Justice and Empowerment supports these services financially. These programmes/services are related to open employment and not to sheltered employment. There is no outcome data available for persons with disabilities placed through NGO sponsored placement agencies.

For self-employment venture, the disabled person also requires support of credit facilities, marketing and support in the form of raw material and land. Banking and financial institutions generally provide various credit facilities. Besides this, District Industrial Centers also give technical advice to entrepreneur wishing to undertake self-employment ventures. But due to lack of marketing skills and confidence, people with disabilities have not utilized these opportunities in formal self-employment ventures. The National Handicapped Finance and Development Corporation, which was established in the year 1997, have special programme for credit facility for self-employment ventures for persons with disabilities and also can act as a catalyst to build confidence among people with disabilities. Besides this, government departments and municipal corporations also provide sites at public places for putting stalls to persons with disabilities on priority basis.[31] Thus in the changing job market scenario, self-employment initiatives have become very important for economic rehabilitation of disabled people.

Under the Ministry of Rural Development, various poverty alleviation programmes is going on the country. Among them Sampoorna Grammeen Rozgar Yojana, Swarnjayanti Gram Swarozgar Yojana, Swarna Jayanti Shahari Rojgar Yojana etc. which focused the persons with disabilities also for empowerment.[32] Although 3 per cent allocation in all the above noted mainstream poverty alleviation programmes are to be made available for disabled persons as per the provisions of 'The Persons with Disabilities (Equal Opportunities, Protection of Rights and Full Participation) Act, 1995, there are no proper mechanisms or procedures established to ensure its compliance. The Government has identified various jobs at different levels for implementing the aforesaid quota scheme. Some of the identified jobs notified by Ministry of Social Justice and Empowerment disability wise are given below.[33] The identified jobs are used for filling up the reservation quota for the respective disability group. Each category of disability is placed against the jobs identified for them to fill up their respective quota in accordance with the scheme of reservation under Section 33 of Persons with Disabilities (Equal Opportunities, Protection of Rights and Full Participation) Act, 1995.

Job opportunities in the open labour market have also been lost by persons with disabilities due to advances in technology. For instance, the jobs of telephone operator and stenography or typist were available to visually impaired but due to change in communication technology and also due to substitution of manual typewriter by computers, these jobs have considerably been reduced. Similarly, since most of the jobs available to persons with disabilities in organized sector were available in government and public sector, globalization has reduced the job opportunities in this sector. The Government has started disinvesting the public sector resulting into reduction of work force in this sector. Unfortunately it has come at a time when private sector was not fully sensitized to the potential of people with disabilities as contributors.

Shortage of appropriate rehabilitation skills is the greatest single problem in developing facilities for disabled persons, and it will take many years to overcome. Two remedies have typically been tried and found wanting: (a) persons who are sent for training; and (b) expatriates are recruited to give training courses (problems include inappropriate course material, inappropriate trainees, and assumption of either administrative or ex-partite posts by trainees). A sharp division is maintained between locally-trained professionals with theoretical knowledge and academic qualifications who devise programs and the hands-on workers. The latter are few and poorly paid. The rehabilitation professionals who have trained and worked may ultimately be the ones who make the system run. They suffer from the disadvantage of being geared to sophisticated systems, and many are naturally prefer to work in western-style "handicap palaces."

Many urge the adoption of low-cost rural community-based schemes at a very modest level of professional skill. The difficulties into which low-cost, community-based schemes are illustrated by the problems of providing primary health care. These include: (a) opposition from professionals and inertia of the status quo; (b) opposition from local communities, who know that if they accept the low-cost scheme they will never get a hospital; (c) difficulty of finding and retaining suitable front-line personnel, maintaining enthusiasm, providing adequate support and supervision, encouragement and some sort of career structure; (d) transport and communication problems; and (e) preference for curative medicine to the near-exclusion of preventive and education measures.

The disability movement in India has long sought to ensure disabled people have guaranteed access to the essential services they need to participate in mainstream society (including education, training and mobility). Arguably economic empowerment is also a question of human rights. When, a government and its international donors place poverty eradication at the heart of public policy, then addressing the economic marginalization of disabled people (who make up one in four of the poor) should have as high a policy priority as primary education or health services.

The disability movement in India will be more sustainable when we will provide proper opportunity to them to develop their capacity. Amartya Sen has argued that capacity building is the key of overall development for any society. For the one of the most backward segment of the society it could be a panacea. For that governmental initiatives is only a drop into the ocean, we all need to contribute our part for the success of empowerment of the disable community. The 2011 census has come with certain positive indicators. But the gravity of the situation demands better vigilance from the government/ civil-society and all other stake holders.

REFERENCES

1. Leandro Despouy, 1993. *Human Right and disabled persons* (study series 6), Centre for Human Rights, UN, Geneva and New York.
2. Peggy Quinn, 1998. *Understanding Disability: a lifespan approach*, Sage Publications, London.
3. Maureen W. Lovett, Feb., 1987. "A Developmental Approach to Reading Disability: Accuracy and Speed Criteria of Normal and Deficient Reading Skill", *Child Development*, Vol. 58, No. 1. pp. 234-260.
4. Serge Resnikoff and Ramachandra Pararajasegaram, 2001, "Blindness prevention programmes: past, present, and future", *Bulletin of the World Health Organization*, 79, pp. 222–226.
5. S. Miles, 1999. *Strenhening Disability and Development Work*, BOND discussion Paper, London, p.7.
6. Ibid. p.15.
7. Ibid. p.17.
8. Janet Seeley, 2001. Recognizing diversity: Disability and Rural livelihoods approaches in India, *Natural Resource Perspectives*, DFID publication by ODI, Vol. 72, October, p.1.
9. DFID, 2000. Disability, Poverty and Development. DFID, London, p.1.
10. Constitutions of India, Directive Principles.
11. Constitutions of India, seventh schedule, list II- state list, entry 9.
12. United Nations, 1994. *The Standard Rules on the Equalisation of Opportunities for Persons with Disabilities*, Disabled Persons Unit,

Department for Policy Co-ordinatlon, United Nations, New York, p.5.

13. See Census 2001.
14. India Country Report, 1999. *Developing an Effective Placement Service for People with Disabilities, Report of a Technical Consultation,* Singapore, p.57.
15. CSO, 2002. NSSO 58th round, Government of India; A comparison of the data of NSSO Surveys of 1981 and 1991 on the magnitude of the problem of disability indicates that the actual number of the disabled has also increased from 136.74 lakhs to 163.62 lakhs and their percentage to the total population in the corresponding years has marginally increased from 1.8 per cent in 1981 to 1.9 per cent in 1991. Amongst the total population of the disabled, persons with locomotor disability had the highest share of 49.2 per cent and the lowest being the victims of speech disability. While the actual number of persons with locomotor disability and visual disability have shown an increasing trend during the last decade (1981-91), persons with hearing disability have shown a decreasing trend; and the persons with speech disability remained more or less the same during the same period. But, when the percentage of their share in the total population of the disabled is considered, all the three categories except for the locomotor disability, have shown a declining trend. The high rate of 49.2 per cent in respect of the persons with locomotor disability was largely attributed to the automobile and road accidents and other industrial hazards, indicating a greater need for strict observation of road and industrial safety measures and traffic regulations.
16. Ministry of Finance, 2004. *Economic Survey, 2003-2004,* Government of India. New Delhi, p. 231.
17. Planning Commission, 2002. *Approach Paper to X Five Year Plan,* Government of India, New Delhi.
18. ILO, March, 2003. *Employment of People with Disabilities: The Impact of Legislation (India Country Profile),* ILO inFocus Programme on Skills, Knowledge and Employability, Development Cooperation Ireland, p. 11.
19. The Ministry of Law and Justice, 1995. *The Persons with Disabilities (equal Opportunities, Protection of rights and Full Participation) act, 1995,* Government of India, New Delhi, p.12.
20. Op. cit. ILO, 2003, p.12.
21. Ibid. p.13.
22. MSJE, 2006. *National Trust Annual Report, 2005-06,* Government of India, New Delhi.p.1; This trust is known for Welfare of Persons with

Autism, Cerebral Palsy, Mental Retardation and Multiple Disabilities under Act, 1999 No. 44 of 1999 (30th December 1999).

23. Ibid. p.7.
24. MSJE, 2004. *Annual Report 2003-2004,* Government of India, New Delhi, p.9.
25. The Persons with Disabilities (equal Opprtunities, protection of rights and Full Participation) Act, 1995, The Chief Commissioner and Commissioners for Persons with Disabilities Chapter XII Section 57, Section 60.
26. Ibid. Chapter II, Section 3.
27. http://www.rehabcouncil.nic.in/council/council.htm
28. Op.cit. MSJE, 2005, p.12.
29. Ministry of Labour, 2006. *Annual Report 2005-06,* Government of India, New Delhi, p. 223.
30. Op.cit. MSJE, p.74.
31. National Handicapped Finance and Development Corporation, 2005. Annual report 2004-05, Government of India, New Delhi, p.5.
32. Ministry of Rural development, *Annual Report 2005-06,* Government of India, New Delhi, p.112.
33. Op.cit. MSJE, p. 2.

Other Sources

DFID, 2000. *Disability: Poverty and Development,* DFID, London

Leandro Despouy, 1993. *Human Right and disabled persons* (study series 6), Centre for Human Rights, UN, Geneva and New York

Mani, D. Rama. *The Physically Handicapped in India: Policy and Programme.* Ashish Publishing House, New Delhi.

Pandey, R., and S. Advani. 1995. *Perspectives in Disable and Rehabilitation,* Vikas Publishing House Pvt. Ltd, New Delhi.

Peggy Quinn, 1998. *Understanding Disability: a lifespan approach,* Sage Publications, London

S. Miles, 1999. *Strenhening Disabiloity and Development Work,* BOND discussion Paper, London.

PART II

DEVELOPMENTAL ISSUES

5

Adjustment Problems of Disabled Children and their Educational Opportunities

Rashmi Sharma and Vandana Bhardawaj

Adjustment is a continuous process by which an individual varies his behaviour to produce a more harmonious relationship between himself and his environment. It is a condition in which the behaviour of an individual conforms to the needs of the individual and demands of the environment. In adjustment, both personal and environmental factors work side by side. An individual is adjusted if he is adjusted to himself and to his environment.

The hearing impairment is one among many physical handicaps of several individuals. It affects adversely the impaired children's performance in learning as it reduces the knowledge of the surrounding environment and the whole world. It develops language inefficiency and reduced communication ability.

It may also become a source of certain adjustment problems as the individuals fail to interact effectively with the people and the environment. Recognizing this, the researcher has undertaken a research study to know about the adjustment problems of the hearing impaired children.

The hearing impaired children are not with much adjustment

problems in home, but are with communication and emotional problems in school. The gender and type of impairment have no effect on adjustment. The children studying in integrated schools have more adjustment problems than the children studying in special schools. In all, the hearing impaired children are enjoying a healthy and supportive life at home and school though there are few adjustment problems.

Human life is the most precious creation of God. It has two aspects – biological and sociological. The biological aspect of human life is maintained and transmitted by nutrition and reproduction. The social aspect of human life is maintained and transmitted by education. Education is considered a vital process in social sense.

Education mainly aims to perfect the individuals in all spheres. Education emphasizes the total development of the individual so that he can make an original contribution to the best of his capacity. Education includes three aspects of the child's development. It should meet, firstly his physical needs, secondly his intellectual needs and thirdly his social and emotional needs.

Education is the key to success in most walks of life. It enlightens the people. It enables the people to know their rights and duties and helps them to secure employment and commands recognition or respect. Lack of education results in problems of sickness, mental ill-health and inadequate child care, thus, leading to much personal unhappiness and frustration for generations together.

Education plays an important role to provide opportunities for the development of the nation. Our constitution has made provision for universal education up to the age of 14 years. All agree that education should reach all children irrespective of their caste, creed and religion. Everybody should get equal opportunities to develop his personality. But, a large number of children are deprived of this privilege. They come under the category of 'Exceptional Children'.

The scheme of Integrated Education for Disabled Children (IEDC) was launched in 1974 to provide educational opportunities for disabled children in the general school system so as to facilitate their retention and integration in the system. Under the scheme 100 per cent financial assistance is provided for education of disabled children which includes assistance towards books and stationery uniforms, transport allowance, readers allowance for blind children, escort allowance for severely handicapped children, boarding and lodging charges for disabled children residing in hostels.

Besides this, assistance is given for setting up and equipping resource rooms with aids and assistive devices, salary of resource teachers, salary of helpers/attendants, funds for survey to identify disabled children, assessment of these children, purchase and production of instructional material, training and orientation of resource teachers, funds for making modifications in the school buildings and the toilets and salary of an Administrative Cell at the State level to implement and monitor the programme.

At present, the IEDC scheme is being implemented in 26 States/ UTs through 14,905 schools. With the coming into force (w.e.f. 7 February 1996) of the Persons with Disabilities Act, 1995, there is now a statutory responsibility on the Central and State government to ensure that all disabled children receive free education in an appropriate environment till the age of 18 years.

Against the allocation of Rs. 21.20 crore, expenditure during the Eighth Plan was Rs. 26.12 crore. For the Ninth Plan period (1997-2002), the scheme of IEDC has projected a budget of Rs. 100 crore with Rs. 13 crore each for the year 1997-98 and 1998-99. The population of disabled children was estimated at 16.15 million whereas the coverage is low. A concerted and coordinated effort is proposed during the Ninth Plan to strengthen the outreach, impact and coverage under the IEDC programme.

Education is the key of empowerment. It makes the way for enlighten and provides an opportunity to the deprived people to get proper amenities for their all round development. Education for all including the person with disabilities, should be treated as a fundamental right, which cannot be realized without their full inclusion. Since inclusion is the focal agenda of the 11th plan therefore it remains of utmost important that persons with disabilities must be educated properly and equal opportunity must be provided to them in this regard. According the working group of disabled constituted by planning commission for the formulation of 11th five year plan "more than 90 per cent disable children and adults have remained out from the educational system.[1] One of the factors behind this is that educational system is not responsive to their needs. According to the report of the working group of disabilities "there is an immediate need to conceptualize an accessible and equitable education framework with the goal of empowering the persons with disabilities. Education, appropriate to the needs of learner, must be viewed as a facilitator of human development of everyone, regardless of status or comparative ability. Moreover, the broad spectrum of individual human capacity to learn must be recognized, and operationalized so that the concepts of special needs and disability become practically manageable in all educational policies and practices."[2]

Growth, development and inclusion all facets of the enhancement of capacity building to the deprived sectors exclusively persons with disabilities could not be achieved till the expansion of education will not be achieved. The 11th five year plan has pointed this issue. Subsequently the government has also enhanced the allocation on education and many varieties of the protection of persons with disabilities has been taken care into the existing framework of education. But due to enormity of the situation, only governmental effort will be merely a drop into the ocean. There is need of charitable actions by all concerned for the proper education of the children with disabilities. Merely governmental arrangements are not going to produce tangible results therefore there is an urgent need to take this issue till its logical conclusion.

REFERENCES

1. Report of the Working Group on Empowering the Disabled for the 11th Five Year Plan, Planning Commission, New Delhi, December 2006, p. 48.
2. *Ibid.*

6

Landmines: The Deadliest Face of Terror, Disability and the United Nations

Vivek Saini

Wars/internal armed conflicts besides natural calamities and accidents, is one of the important reasons of human disability. Among various weapons which cause terrible injuries mutilation leading of disability, landmines is the foremost one. Anti-personnel landmines (APL), the improved version of landmine, because of their deadly and deceptive power of destruction, killing and maimings are rightly described as "silent and deceptive burried terror beneath the earth" and "weapons of mass destruction and misery in slow motion."[1] Landmines were firstly seen during the American civil war (1860-65). They were further developed and used during the World War I known as Anti-Tank Mines (ATM), mainly to destroy or incapacitate the advancing tanks and other armoured and non-armoured vehicles of the enemy. Later they were further developed and converted into the APL, mainly designed as defensive weapons to impede the enemy's advance.

Today millions of landmines are scattered in some 78 countries causing around 26,000 million deaths or injuries ever year.[2] Landmines are more deadly and dangerous compared to other conventional weapons. They, unlike other weapons of war most of which are aimed and fired towards enemy, the anti-personnel landmines are victim actuated that is they are designed to be detonated by a person stepping on or handling the device, or by accidentally disturbing trip wire attacked to it. Once coming into contact with a human being with some pressure, there occurs loud explosion and the victim mostly losses one or two limbs or losses life. Hence APM makes no distinction between friends or foe, unarmed civilian and a belligerent. Whosoever comes into its contact, is either killed or maimed permanently. So innocent children playing or civilians going about his or her daily activities become its unfortunate victims. The destructive power of APM continues for indefinite period. The APMs planted during the Vietnam War in Vietnam, Cambodia and Laos continue killing and maiming the innocent citizens even today.

While all war wounds and injuries are severe, the injuries inflicted by anti-personnel mines are particularly horrific. Because the APMs are designed to kill, and more often, to disable their victims permanently. They are specifically constructed to shatter limits beyond repair. The detonation of a burried APM blasts rips off one or both legs of the victims. Moreover the APM drives soil, grass, gravel, dust metal, the plastic fragments and explosive material in to the muscles of the lower part of the body. Thus, in addition to the severe injuries, there is threat of serious infection. In addition to amputation of the limbs, gangarine reaches other parts of the body leading to the loss of more limbs. Treating of a mine-injured patient is a serious challenge to the most competent surgeon. While the reality is that most of the mine victims are extremely poor living in countries with extremely limited medical and rehabilitation resources. Their access to proper treatment, care and rehabilitation is thus difficult or impossible. Since World War II, landmines have severely injured and permanently disabled more people, combatants and civilians alike both, than any other weapons.

The APM, besides its severe destructive power is very cheap and easy to plant. Hence the APMs are used not only by the military in the wars. But also by insurgents and terrorists in villages, fields, forests, river beds and roads etc. Due to this, millions of acres of taxed agricultural land have become unfit for cultivation. The presence of landmines leaves large portion of the national territory unfit for any kind of use. Farmland, grazing pastures and other food producing areas are rendered inaccessible and as a result, the ability of a community to feed itself is impaired. Mined roads, and railway make the movement of persons and goods, including delivery of humanitarian aid, extremely difficult. Because of the APMs, people have to leave their fields and homes and migrate to other places during peace time making them internally displaced persons. In this way the APMs not only disabled the people but uproot them from their home and deprive them of their fundamental right to live and earn their livelihood peacefully.

Mine clearance, although essential, but is very expensive, slow and dangerous process. While planting a mine costs only 3 to 4 dollar, but to demine and defuse it cost from $300 to $1000.[3] Thus the cost of demining the world (estimates more than 150 million of 78 countries) would be from $10 billion to $110 billion. According to an United Nations estimate more than 150 million APMs are in storage and than 2 to 2.5 millions mines are laid every year. While only 500,000 are located and destroyed in a year.[4] In this way it would take more than one thousand years to free the world from the landmines.

The unrestricted use of landmines is prohibited under the principles of international law. There are two major sources of international law. First is the General International Humanitarian Law, and second is the Treaty Law. Under the former come the Hague Convention (18 October, 1907) and the Geneva Convention (1949) and its Additional Protocol I (1977). Article 23(c) of the Convention prohibits "the use of such weapons and projectiles which cause unnecessary or superfluous suffering."[5] This means that any weapon designed to cause more injury than required even to a soldier i.e. one intended to inflict unnecessary suffering, is unlawful and must not be used under the Hague Convention 1907. Article 25 of this Convention directs that cities, villages, buildings and other human habitants should not be made target. Hence practices to conflicts must always distinguish between civilians and the combatants and civilians must not be the subject to attack. In accordance with this rule, any weapon that is inherently and indiscriminately killed or injured must never be used. Similarly, Additional Protocol I (1997) of the Geneva Convention 1949 under article 51 directs that the population of citizens which are non-combatants must be saved from indiscriminate attacks in all circumstances. Article 51(b) prohibits the use of such weapons which cause more and unnecessary bodily suffering compared to the legitimate military objectives.[6] The careful study of these various principles of the international humanitarian law reveal that the landmines, which do not discriminate between the soldiers and civilians and cause unnecessary, superfluous and severe suffering come under their prohibition.

These rules of international humanitarian law are universally applicable to all states whether they have become parties to these conventions or not. Besides, there are Treaty Laws, which are applicable only to those states who have ratified them. To control the unrestricted use of landmines, the United Nations adopted the Convention on Certain Conventional Weapons (CCW) in 1980, the full title of which is the "United Nation's Convention on Prohibitions or Restrictions on the use of Certain Conventional Weapons which may be deemed to be excessively injurious or to hence indiscriminate effects."[7]

As the civilian impact of the landmines became more and more serious, it was apparent that the existing provisions of the UN Convention on Certain Conventional Weapons (1980) were too weak and were not adequately followed by many countries where mines were being freely used. Following a formal request by France in 1993, governments agreed to meet and review this UN Convention on Certain Conventional Weapons and strengthen it. The result was that Protocol II to the Convention strengthening restrictions on certain uses transfers, and types (self-destroying and detectable) of landmines was adopted (on 1998) by the United Nations. The main provisions of the Protocol II to the CCW Convention are as follows:

I. Mines may be directed only at military objectives. Their indiscriminate use is prohibited, and all feasible precautions must be taken to protect the civilians.
II. Remotely delivered mines should not be used unless these

locations are accurately recorded in the specific register and each landmines is fitted with an effective self-neutralizing mechanism.

III. Proper records must be kept of the location of pre-planted mine-fields, and parties to the conflict should endeavour to keep record of the location of each mine field laid during hostilities. Each party to the conflict would provide this information to the other parties to the conflict after the hostilities are over.

IV. At the end of the hostilities the parties are to try to agree both among themselves and with other effective states and organizations to take necessary effective measures to clear the mine-fields.

This Protocol II to the CCW too was weak and ineffective. Its greatest loophole was that it applied only with regard to the conflicts between states only. Originally it did not apply to the internal armed conflicts where the non-state actors, the terrorists and other extremist groups use landmines and consequently numerous lives are lost.

Here the United Nations stepped in and played vital role. The UN Secretary General Boutrous Ghali appointed a Group of Governmental Experts to look into the matter. The Group met several times during 1994-95 and suggested the amendment to the Protocol II of the 1980 Convention on Excessively Injurious Conventional Weapons. The amended Protocol was to be extended to internal strifes and put ban on transfer of such weapons to the non-state entities.

The United Nations continued addressing the problem posed by the landmines. In early November 1996 the United States and eighty four co-sponsor states submitted a draft resolution to the UN General Assembly to "pursue vigorously an effective, legally binding ban" has on the use, stockpiling, production and transfer of APMs, calling on all states to accede to the CCW and its amended Protocol II, to comply to the fullest extent possible with the applicable rules of the Protocol, and to declare and implement various moratoria, bans and other restrictions on landmines already announced by other states. The resolution was approved in the First Committee of General

Assembly on 13 November 1996 by a vote of 141 in favour, none against it, with 10 abstentions (Belarus China, Cuba, North Korea, South Korea, Israel, Pakistan, Russia, Syria and Turkey). The states abstaining the resolution took the stand that mines were legitimate means of self-defence and national security. Russian representative stated that solidarity with victims of landmine should be expressed through intensification of mine cleaning efforts and a ban on the export rather than on the use and production of mines. The representative of China said that the right to self-defence must be taken in to account while opposing the production and use of landmines.

On 10 December 1996, the UN General Assembly adopted the important resolution (GA Res. 51/45S). The resolution[8] requested the Secretary-General to prepare a report on steps taken to complete in international agreement banning the use, stock-piling, production and transfer of APMs, and on other steps taken by member states to implement such bans, moratoria or other restrictions and to submit it to the General Assembly all its fifty-second session. The resolution further called upon all states to support a new international agreement totally prohibiting anti-personnel mines "as soon as possible". A total number of 157 countries voted in favour of this resolution, none opposed it and only 10 abstained from voting.

Later at the first review conference, an amendment to Protocol II to the Convention was agreed upon whereby the amended Protocol II of the Convention now applies to both internal conflicts as well as conflicts between states. The amended Protocol II of the Convention entered in to force on 3 December 1998. As of June, 2007, 86 states including India have become parties to the Protocol II of the UN CCW Convention of 1980.[9] Under this revised and amended Protocol to the CCW Convention, the States parties agree (a) never to use such weapons covered by the Protocol II if they are of a nature to cause unnecessary suffering or superfluous injuries, (b) never to use those weapons if they are designed to explode under the effect of mine detection equipment; (c) never to direct these weapons against civilians or civilian objects; and (d) never to use these weapons indiscriminately.[10]

In this way this amended Protocol II too could not impose total ban on the use of landmines. It too however put certain restrictions. But its provisions were extremely complex and many member states doubted whether they could be effectively implemented in most situations of internal armed conflicts. Only few believed that the amended Protocol would be sufficient to reduce the number of civilian's landmines casualties.[11]

Now the group of like-minded and pro-ban countries like Norway, Germany, Belgium, Austria, Japan, Germany and Canada with the active support of many organizations and agencies emerged and accelerated their efforts in the direction of producing the total ban Convention. The Canada sponsored strategy conference Towards a Gloha Ban on Anti-Personnel Mines, took place in Ottawa in October 1996 with the active support of 50 governments, the International Committee of Red Cross (ICRC) the International Campaign to Ban Landmines (ICBL) and the United Nations. On 5 October 1996, the conference adopted the Ottawa Declaration, which committed the participants to carrying out a plan of action intended to increase resources and to working to ensure that a ban treaty was to be concluded at the earliest possible date. At the closing of the conference the Canadian government invited all governments to come to Ottawa in December 1997 to sign a comprehensive anti-landmines treaty.

The international support for the ban on landmines continued to grow. To support the Ottawa process, the Austrian government prepared a draft text of the ban treaty and circulated it to the interested governments and organizations. This Austrian draft which was subsequently revised a number of times was the basis of the ban treaty concluded in Oslo in September 1997. International discussion on the draft text began had already begun in Vienna in February 1997 at the meeting hosted by the Austrian government. In its address to the meeting the ICRC called for a comprehensive ban treaty based on a unambiguous definition of an anti-personnel mine. In April 1997, the German Government hosted a special meeting to discuss possible verification measures to be included in the total ban treaty.

The formal follow-up to the 1996 Ottawa conference took place in Brussels from 24-27 June 1997. The Brussels International Conference for a Global Ban on Anti-Personnel Mines was attended by representatives of 154 countries. It was the largest gathering of governments to date for a conference devoted specifically to the issue of banning landmines. On the closing day 97 governments signed the Brussels Declaration, launching formal negotiations on a comprehensive landmine ban treaty, greater international cooperation and assistance for nine clearance and the destruction of all stockpiled and cleared anti-personnel mines. The Brussels Declaration called for the convening of a diplomatic conference in Oslo to negotiate such a treaty on the basis of the draft prepared by the Austrian government.

In accordance with the Brussels Declaration, which by now have been signed by 107 countries, formal treaty negotiations took place from 1 to 18 September 1997 at the Oslo Diplomatic Conference on an International Total Ban on Anti-Personnel Land Mines, hosted by the Norwegian government. Ninety one countries took part in the negotiations as full participants and 38 countries were present as observers, as were the ICRC, ICBL and the United Nations.

The Oslo Diplomatic Conference proved to be a tremendous successful and paved the way to the Ottawa Conference where the most important international Anti-Personnel Mines Ban Convention (APMBC) was adopted on 1 March 1999. Also known as the Ottawa Convention, it is officially referred to as the "Convention on the Prohibition of the Use, Stockpiling, Production and Transfer of Anti-Personnel Mines and Their Destruction". It imposes a total ban on anti-personnel landmines.[12] The state parties to the Ottawa Convention undertook obligations:

(a) Never to use, develop, produce, stockpile, or transfer anti-personnel landmines or to assist any other party to conduct these activities.
(b) To destroy all stockpiled anti-personnel landmines within four years of the convention entry in to force.
(c) When it is within their measures, to provide assistance to mine clearance mine awareness, stockpile destruction, and victims assistance activities world wide.
(d) State parties to the Ottawa Convention also agree to report annually to the UN Secretary-General on: (i) national

measures to implement the Convention; (ii) their stockpiles of anti-personnel landmines; (iii) the location of mines areas within country; (iv) landmines They retain for training purpose; (v) progress achieved in mines clearance and stockpiles; (vi) destruction of the number of landmines and the types of landmines destroyed; (vii) progress achieved in decommissioning production facilities for landmines; (viii) measures taken to protect the civilian population from anti-personnel landmines in the country.

As of August 2007, 155 states had become parties to the Ottawa Convention.[13]

But there are many countries, particularly India, China and Pakistan from the South Asian region who have not yet put their signatures, not to speak of ratifying the Ottawa Convention. They feel that landmines are very cheap and effective measures to tackle the internal armed conflicts and protect the borders against incursions. Hence they are not in favour of immediate and total ban on the use of landmines. They want gradual and partial prohibition, and while doing so, their security concerns should be well taken care of. Many countries like Russia, USA, China and many East European countries manufacture and export landmines. The total ban would adversely affect their economic interest. Thus because of their selfish economic interests they do not favour the total ban of landmines. The seriousness of the issue demands that, keeping aside their own selfish interests all the countries should lend their full support to the total ban on the production, stockpile, export, import and use of landmines. The use of APMs should be totally prohibited in the armed conflicts between states as well in internal armed conflicts between non-state actors.

United Nation's Role in the Field of Demining and Rehabilitation of Mines Victims

On ground, 14 agencies, programmes, departments and funds are active in mine-related service in about 71 mines affected countries of the world. They find and destroy landmines, assist victims of landmines in several ways and teach people how to remain safe in mine affected areas. Thus the core elements of UN mine action programme[14] are:

(i) Minefield Survey;
(ii) Mapping of the mine fields;
(iii) Marking of the mines burried underneath;
(iv) Clearance and demining;
(v) Assistance to the victims including rehabilitation and reintegration in the society.

The United Nations Mine Action Service (UNMAS) coordinates all mine-related activities in the UN System. It develops policies and standards, conduct ongoing assessment and monitoring of the threat posed by mines, collects and disseminates information, mobilizes resources and engages in advocacy in support of the global ban on anti-personnel landmines. It is also responsible for the provision of mine-action assistance in humanitarian agencies and for peace keeping operations. UNMAS activities are not funded by the regular UN budget but supported through the Voluntary Trust Fund to Assistance in Mine Action, and by the contribution of the donor countries.

One of the UNMAS main responsibilities is to assess and monitor the global landmine threat, to identify needs, and to make appropriate responses to those needs. It has sent its several missions to Azerbajan, Burundi, Ethopia, Somalia, Yemen, Jordan and Lebanon. The aim of these missions was to define the scope and nature of the landmines problems in the affected countries, to identify constrains and opportunities relating to the development of mine-action initiatives and to make recommendations for a comprehensive responses, including institutional arrangements for the coordination and implementation of mine action activities. The programme and activities of UNMAS were undertaken in Angola, Bosnia and Herzegovina, Croatia Cambodia, Lao, Mozambique Afghanistan with the financial assistance of UNDP.[15]

The UN Mine Action Programme for Afghanistan (MAPA)[16]

The UN Mine Action Programme for Afghanistan (MAPA) is one

of the world's largest civilian mine clearance programme. It is carried out through following means.

1. Manual Mines clearance;
2. Mechanical Mines clearance;
3. Mines Detection Dogs;
4. Battle Areas clearance;
5. Explosive ordinance disposal.

This programme focuses on mine survey, mapping of mine fields, marking mines and then demining. The MAPA also provides mine risk education and comprehensive training in mine detection and mine clearance. For the first time it introduced in the large scale mine detection dogs squad in the world. The programme focuses on the development of indigenous capacity to respond to the problem of demining by creating the indigenous NGOs. Thus MAPA on the one hand achieves indigenous partnership in demining, on the other hand it provides employment to the unemployed persons of the affected country. Thus, it has become a vehicle of development.

Mine Clearance Planning Agency (MCPA)[17]

Another important indigenous non-governmental organization which is an implementing partner of MAPA in MCPA. It has undertaken the task of mine field surveys, mine clearance surveys, battle area surveys, and socio-economic surveys. It operates with 31 survey teams and one rapid response survey team. Each MCPA survey team consists of five-members. All survey teams are trained in battle area survey technique. The survey output is used by all nine-clearance organizations. Since its establishment in Afghanistan MCPA survey teams identified, marked, mapped and recorded more than 680 million square meters of mines contaminated areas and have cleared about 68 million square meters of suspected mines infested area and has destroyed 6,335 anti-personnel mines and 680 anti-tank mines and 11,366 UXO. MCPA maintains comprehensive computerized information system for the mine action. It has developed its own data base and a computerized mapping system. Its computerized information system has played a vital role in the mine clearance action operations.

Monitoring Education and Training Agency (META)

The UN office for the Coordination of Humanitarian Assistance to Afghanistan set up META to monitor and evaluate the efficiency and effectiveness of mine action programme. The key goals of META as suggested by UNOCHA[18] are to:

(a) Provide high quality training in mine clearance skills and techniques;
(b) Conduct monitoring to ensure safety and implementation of standard operation Procedures (SOPs);
(c) Investigate demining accidents to identify the causes and to suggest the remedial measures;
(d) Provide support to the research and development activities of MAPA;
(e) Maintain mine clearance manual and record.

As a monitoring body, META monitors all mine action teams, battle area clearance and make survey at least twice a year. During 2006 the META conducted 240 monitoring missions. It also arranged investigations of cases of poor performance in mine clearance. META provides training programmes in the field of mine detection, copying and clearance. It offers various types of courses to the deminers which involves individual training, group training refresher training safety related training and battle area clearance courses. META also offers management and monitoring course. META makes accidents investigations to find out the factors for leading to accidents and suggest preventive measures so that accidents are not repeated. META finally checks and clears all land after demining and removal of land mines before it is handed over to the community. As such META finally inspects the previously demined mines areas before declaring it safe for use. So it takes absolutely no chance of mine blasts during its use in future.

Mine De ion and Dog Centre (MDC)[19]

MDC also functions under the supervision of the UN Mine Action Programme for Afghanistan (MAPA) and is financially supported by the UN Mine Action Centre for Afghanistan (MACA) and other donor countries like Japan, Germany, and Norway Canada etc. MDA works for mine clearance with the help of Mine Dog Groups (MDGs). The trained dogs work very fast and efficiently in the field of mine clearance. So MDGs immensely increase the mine clearance with little chance of human accidents. An MDG is able to clear 2000 to 5000 sq. m. per day. Since 2005 MDG have cleared, 82,338 sq. m. area Currently MDG deploys 68 mine Dog Groups for mine clearance operations and 59 Mine Dog Sets (MDSs) for mine survey operation in different parts of Afghanistan.[20]

UN Activities in the Field of Rehabilitation

The United Nations in cooperation with other international bodies like the International Committee of the Red Cross (ICRC) plays very important role in rehabilitating the mine victims. It has set up many hospitals and orthopedic centers where mine victims are freely treated and amputees are provided artificial limbs. The ICRC with the financial assistance from UNDP operate 50 projects in 22 countries which manufacture millions of artificial limbs for the amputees. They also make orthoses, a device which supports a paralyzed limb, crutches and wheel chairs. These are given free to the mine victims. The ICRC's projects provides training to the local technicians. The aim of the ICRC is to provide immediate relief to those mine victims who need rehabilitation. To ensure sustainability, the ICRC approach emphasises on the use of locality available resources and expertise so that the rehabilitation programmes become technically self-sufficient. Artificial limbs and support systems are made using locally available steel, wood, leather and other materials with indigenous expertise. But at the same time research work continues to make them light weight, comfortable and long lasting.[21] For example "Jaipur foot" of India weighting about 1 Kg, made of rubber resin, aluminum and leather is comfortable, durable, and waterproof and can be worn without a shoe. It is used by the mine victims of the Aro-Asian countries.

Physical rehabilitation programmes run by the United Nations and other international agencies is only a part of the solution to reduce the suffering and disability caused by the landmines. The ultimate aim is to improve the quality of life of the mine-victims and to enable them to once again fully participate in their communities. More importantly, efforts to impose legal binding, immediate, absolute and complete ban on the use, stockpiling, production and transfer, of all anti-personnel mines must be relentlessly pursued. Only such a comprehensive, and not a piece-meal approach will succeed in ridding the world of this cruel and dreadful weapon which has mutilated and disabled more and more people in the war as well as peace time than any other weapon.

REFERENCES

1. Michael J. Matheson, "New Landmines Protocol: Vital Step towards its Ban", in *Arms Control Today* (Geneva), 10 July 1998, p.10.
2. *The United Nations Today* (New Look: UN Dept of Public Information, 2008), p. 141.
3. Christopher S Ray ed. *Stalking Terror: Landmines in Peace and in War* (Delhi Words Miths, 2000), p. 16.
4. *UN/DIR, New Letter,* "The Elimination of Landmines: Special Issue" (Geneva, 2002), p. 30.
5. *International Committee Red Cross* (ICRC) "The Geneva Convention of 12 August 1949: Commentary III (Geneva, Convention Relating to the Treatment of Prisoners of War" (Geneva, 1960), pp. 130-31.
6. ICRC, *Commentary on the Additional Protocols to the Geneva Convention of 12* August, 1949, (Geneva, 1987), p. 613.
7. *For Text of the Convention* see "Year book of the United Nations 1980", Vol. 34 (New York: UN Department of Public Information, 1983), pp. 76-77.
8. For Text of the resolution, see *Year book of the United Nations 1996,* Vol.50 (New York UN Department of Public Information, 1998), pp. 482-83.
9. *The United Nations Today* (New York: UN Department of Public Information, 2008), p. 139.
10. For more details see, *Year book of the United Nations,* 1998, Vol. 52, (New York, 2001), pp. 536-37.
11. ICRC, *Banning Anti-Personnel Mines* (Geneva, 1998), p. 3.
12. For Text of the Ottawa Convention 1999 see ICRC, *Banning Anti-Personnel Mines: The Ottawa Treaty Explained,* Geneva, 1998), Annexure, 11, pp. 14-20.

13. *The United Nations Today* (New York, Department of Public Information, 2008), p. 139.
14. For details see, *U.N. Landmines: A Special Issue, A review of United Nations Activities in Mine Action* (Geneva, 2006), pp. 36-39.
15. Ibid.
16. For details see United Nations, *Mine Action Programme in Afghanistan: A Continuing Challenge* (Special Issues) July 2002, New York, 2002.
17. For details about MCPA, see *MCPA; Socio-Economic Impact: Study of Mine Action Operations: Afghanistan.* Interim Report by MCPA to United Nations, October 2001.
18. For details See *U.N., Landmines: A Review of United Nations Activities in Mine Action CA special issue,* New York, 2001.
19. *UN Landmines: A special Issue, op. cit.* no.14
20. *UN Mine Action Progamme in Afghanistan, op. cit.* 16.
21. *UN Landmines* (Geneva, 2004).

7

Protecting Rights of Disabled: An Educational Intervention

Jayadeba Sahoo

In this threshold of a new millennium, today we are witnessing the familiar patterns of genocides, mass murders, and massive violations of human rights caused by the rise of racism, xenophobia, sexism and religious intolerance that tear people apart within nations. Certainly, cold war has come to a close. Still, no less disturbing for the protection of human rights, world peace, and security are new threats stemming from environmental degradation, terrorism, biomedical tech., drug addiction and HIV/AIDS. The scourge is universal.

Thus 'if we want to preserve this humanity, we must give every chance to peace, freedom and conviviality. Because lasting peace is a prerequisite for the exercise of all human rights and duties,' says Federico Mayor, the Director General of UNESCO.

So there is talk of human rights. Human rights as a global phenomenon are inherent in nature, which refers to fundamental freedom and basic liberties without which one cannot live with peace, happiness, respect and dignity. The idea that there are equal rights for everybody and freedoms that apply to everybody is an idea of modern times. This idea of Human Rights first emerged with the Megna Carta of 1215 and the Bill of Rights and 1689 in England and spread with the Declaration of Independence of the USA in 1776 and the Declaration of Rights of Man and the Citizens in France in 1789, but the idea of Human Rights only really took place on a Universal dimension with the adaptation by the UN General Assembly of the Universal Declaration of Human Rights (UDHR) in 10th December, 1948.

Later two more documents were adopted namely:

(a) International covenants on Economic, Social and Cultural Rights (ICESCR) and its optional Protocol.
(b) International Covenant on Civil and Political Rights (ICCP) and its optional Protocol.

These three documents together constitute the International Bill of Human Rights.

India is a multi-cultural, multi-ethnic, multi-religious and multi-linguistic society and persons of all faiths and beliefs live together. However, there are some disparities in services to persons belonging to specific groups. Disability is one such area which has experienced low priority in the service sector. It is important that we first become aware of the Conceptual/definitional aspects of the area of disability.

Impairment, Disability, Handicap

The terminologies like impairment, disability and handicap ate interchangeably used by professionals, though there is a change in the philosophical and sociologic interpretations of these terms. These interpretations are made on the basis of the extent of disability in the individual. However, these differences in terminologies also provide opportunities for their discrimination in the society.

Impairment means damage to the tissues. It can be measured and cured and it does not impose obstacles to a larger extent with any of the social and vocational pursuits of the individual. By knowing the limitations the impairment may impose, a person can take all measures to compensate or even to ignore it for his/her normal functioning.

Disability indicates the permanent loss of the functions of the particular organ to the extent that the individual cannot fully participate in the social and vocational pursuits. But this condition does not prevent the individual from overcoming his/her disability condition and from using his/her skills to the optimum level possible. When the ability aspect of the individual is focused, the disability disappears to a large extent.

Disability is generally defined as any restriction or lack (resulting from impairment) of ability to perform an activity in the manner or within the range considered as normal for a human being. According to the United Nations, disabled persons are those who are unable to ensure themselves, wholly or partly, the necessities of a normal individual and/or social life, as a result of a deficiency, either congenital or not, in their physical or mental capabilities; or persons with restrictions or lack of ability to perform an activity in the manner or within the range considered normal for a human being. A disability becomes a handicap when it interferes with one's ability to do what is expected at a particular time.

Handicap is made and not acquired. Discrimination on the basis of disability leads to the handicapping condition. The disability surrounded by a distressing environment makes the person a handicap. Disabled individuals who live in the most restrictive environment experience handicapping conditions.

The need for non-discrimination should be taught to young children so that the disability does not become a handicap. As experienced by Helen Keller and others, the attitude of the public towards disability condition is the hardest burden to bear. Sometimes it is stereotypic in nature.

Categories of Disabilities

Disabled are of two broad categories: physical and mental. The physically disabled include the deaf, dumb, blind and orthopedics. Mental disability includes mental retardation, autism and cerebral palsy. According to the Persons With Disabilities (Equal Opportunities, Protection of Rights and Full Participation) (PWD) Act, 1995, seven categories of disabilities have been included under disability like, blindness, low vision, leprosy-cured, hearing impairment, locomotor disability, mental retardation, and mental illness. These disabilities have been further defined in the Act as:

(a) "Blindness" refers to a condition where a person suffers from any of the following conditions, namely:

  (i) total absence of sight; or
  (ii) visual acuity not exceeding 6/60 or 20/200 (snellen) in the better eye with correcting lenses; or
  (iii) limitation of the field of vision subtending an angle of 20 degrees or worse

(b) "Person with Low Vision" means a person with impairment of visual functioning even after treatment or standard refractive correction but who uses or is potentially capable of using vision for the planning or execution of a task with appropriate assistive devices.

    WHO (1992) defines that a person with low vision is one who has impairment of visual functioning even after treatment and/or standard refractive correction, and has a visual acuity of less than 6/18 to light perception or a visual field of less than 10 degrees from the point of fixations, but who uses, or is potentially able to use vision for the planning or execution of a task.

(c) "Hearing impairment" means loss of sixty decibels or more in the better ear in the conversational range of frequencies. "Mental retardation" means a condition of arrested or incomplete development of mind of a person which is specially characterised by subnormality of intelligence.

(d) Mental retardation simply means that the person with mental retardation will have the Intelligence Quotient (IQ) of less than 70. In addition to the low IQ, there will also be problems for these children in performing daily living skills.

(e) "Mental illness" means any mental disorder other than mental retardation

(f) "Locomotor disability" means disability of the bones, joints or muscles leading to substantial restriction of the movement of the limbs or any form of cerebral palsy.

(g) "Leprosy cured person" means any person who has been cured of leprosy but is suffering from:

(i) loss of sensation in hands or feet as well as loss of sensation and paresis in the eye and eye-lid but with no manifest deformity
(ii) manifest deformity and paresis but having sufficient mobility in their hand and feet to enable them to engage in normal economic activity
(iii) extreme physical deformity as well as advanced age which prevents him/her from undertaking any gainful occupation.

Other Disabilities

Though the PWD Act defines only the above categories of disabilities, children with other disabilities are also in need of educational services. For example, learning disability is one category. Children with learning disabilities are those who have problems in processing information. "Cerebral palsy" is another category and means a group of non-progressive conditions of a person characterised by abnormal motor control posture resulting from brain insult or injuries occurring in the pre-natal, peri-natal or infant period of development. Children with multiple disabilities have also not been included in the Act. However, these children have to be given educational services, when identified.

When the child exhibits a combination of the above disabilities, the problem would multiply further. Provision of education may be possible for those children with multiple disabilities whose cognitive functions are in order whereas only limited education and rehabilitation services can be planned for those whose cognitive functions are defective. For example, educational programmes can be planned for a blind child with hearing impairment or locomotor disability whereas a blind child with mental retardation may find education extremely difficult. Therefore, individual assessment is imperative for planning appropriate educational programmes for these children.

Disabilities: Imbalances and Discriminatory Practices

Disability is one such area which has experienced low priority in the service sector. The reasons for the low priority can be attributed to many factors. As inclusion of persons with disabilities in the society becomes vital to empower them with human rights, certain positive measures should be initiated at all levels to overcome the present imbalances and discriminatory practices. The concept of inclusive society centres around three issues, namely—cultures, policies and practices.

In terms of culture, India remains a united country, despite its diversities, and a person with disability is not isolated just for the reason that he/she is disabled. We learn from history that disabled persons during the Spartan days were even destroyed. The attitude of destruction slowly changed as a symbol of punishment in the society. These extreme attitudes were not present in India even in the past. Though there is a 'Karma' Theory in India which conceptualizes that what we are today is because of the result of the past lives, there was no attitude of destruction of persons with disabilities. In ancient India, social orders were initiated in pre- and Vedic times and those were in tune with the natural order. Persons with disabilities were accepted as part of that natural order and were accommodated and adjusted to daily life activities of those times.

The first school for the deaf and the blind were started in India in 1884 and 1887 respectively, though disabled persons lived even before that time. There was social inclusion of these persons in the society even then. The discrimination started in provisions of the tangible practices, as in India, more than 90 per cent of persons with disabilities, most of whom live in rural areas, do not have access to any services but they are not isolated from the communities. They live in the society but their needs are not addressed. This condition may be called as social inclusion.

In terms of practices, the main problem in the country is with respect to their actualization. Discrimination is experienced only in terms of actual services extended to persons with disabilities.

At the national level, there is no authentic survey to provide information on the number of disabled children who are in need of services. Many surveys made in the past were based on sample surveys and they differed in using the definitions to a large extent. Mander and Rao (1996) mention that there is limited information regarding the actual extent and range of prevalence of the disability and, therefore, to find out the actual number, one may wish to comprehensively cover, possibly a district or some administrative segment of a district.

The only national level project which made a door-to-door survey of disabled children in the entire block was the Project Integrated Education for the Disabled (PIED) supported by UNICEF through NCERT from 1987 to 1993. The project was implemented in one representative block in each of the States namely, Rajasthan (Chabbra block), Madhya Pradesh (Masturi), Maharashtra (Palghar), Orissa (Baliantha), Tamil Nadu (Kattankulathur), Nagaland (Kikruma), Mizoram (Khazal), Haryana (Bhiwani), and the Municipal Corporations Delhi (Trans-Yamuna) and Baroda. The disabled children identified in these blocks are indicated in Table 1.

Table 1: Prevalence of Children with Disabilities

S. No.	Block	Blind Deaf	Mentally Retarded	Locomotor	Handicapped
1.	Chhabra	113	278	76	436
2.	Masturi	124	126	29	679
3.	Palghar	48	100	39	118
4.	Baliantha	51	110	72	95
5.	Kattanku lathur	52	95	84	224
6.	Kikruma	53	77	19	63
7.	Khazal	67	108	83	68
8.	Bhiwani	99	123	64	543
9.	Trans- Yamuna	63	88	90	257
10.	Baroda MC	108	131	99	157

Note: The statistics obtained out of this project can be projected safely as this is the only survey conducted on the basis of' 'Whole block approach'. As per the PIED, nearly 2.5 per cent of the children of school going population have disability of some kind.

Approaches in Identifying Children with Disabilities

The manpower development document of the Rehabilitation Council of India (RCI) (1995) reports that not even five per cent of the disabled population is currently enjoying educational facilities. The reason is that the present educational system is not able to take education to the doorsteps of the children. To provide education to this uncovered population, appropriate strategies need to be adopted for locating them for early intervention services. Early intervention would solve many of the problems of the child later in life. While early identification is of paramount importance in the life of every child, it is more vital in the case of children with disabilities. Research studies indicate that the children identified and provided services early in life find integration in the community natural, real and effective.

As evident from the definitions of various disability conditions, some persons experience difficulties in cognitive functions, some in senses and some others in their physical and bodily conditions. The common approaches in identifying persons with disabilities are as follows:

(a) **Cognitive approach:** By adopting the cognitive approach, identification of children may be made as those who are mentally retarded, slow learners, normal learners, academically advanced learners and gifted learners. This identification is purely based on the cognitive functions of the child. For example:

- The child who has an IQ between 50 and 75 will come under the category of educable mentally retarded child.
- The trainable mentally retarded children have an IQ of 25 to 50 and they may find it difficult even to perform manual kind of work.
- Those who have an IQ of less than 25 are called totally dependent category.

In developed countries, not only children with mental retardation, but also children having slow learning skills are also given special attention. For example, slow learners but not mentally retarded children, and academically advanced learners but not gifted are given special opportunities to manifest their abilities. However, the Indian condition is different. Most of the children who have non-observable disability conditions are already absorbed in the system. They are not labelled as children with disabilities. For example, children having IQ range of 70-130 are found in the general classrooms. This is a blessing in disguise. Sometimes, the learning needs of these children go unnoticed and as a result, they become dropouts from the system. On the other hand, their self-esteem is intact as they are not labelled as disabled children. Of the two, non-labeling has a positive impact on the individual and, therefore, it is better if these children are not labelled as children with disabilities. In order to help them, it is vital to improve the abilities of general classroom teachers to teach children of all categories. Innovative teachers always take care of children with different intellectual abilities. Therefore, the onus lies on the quality of general teacher preparation centres.

(b) **Sensory approach:** Through sensory approach, visually impaired, hearing impaired and deaf-blind children can be identified. Out of them, visually impaired children are neither cognitive impaired nor communication impaired. They lack abilities in the orientation of environment. The mobility skills are also affected due to the loss of vision. On the other hand, the deaf child's main problem is in the area of communication skills. Some of them use lip-reading skills whereas some use sign language. It is proper to use total communication system, which uses the combination of both. The deaf-blind children will have a serious disadvantage in both orientation and communication skills. As a result, these children have to be provided compensatory experiences mostly through tactile approach. As blind and deaf children are not impaired cognitively, they can follow the same curriculum meant for the sighted and hearing children. However, certain curricular adaptations have to be made to suit their learning styles.

(c) **Ability-based approach:** There are many children who experience difficulty in processing information. Though their intelligence is normal and senses, too, are normal, sometimes they perform poorly due to Jack of ability in processing information. Information processing theorists feel that these children lack adequate skills in attention, perception, memory, encoding etc. These children are called as learning disabled children. Dysgraphia, Dyslexia and Dyscalculia are some of the defects associated with the learning problems in general. Research indicates that these children can also be made to learn through specific modality approaches such as improving attention skills, perceptual abilities, etc.

(d) **Society-based approach:** Among disabled children, some of them are facing emotional problems too. The behaviour disorders in these children may also be a result of social problems such as the state of experience of neglect, over-protection, etc. A disabled child who doesn't have a conducive family support or parental affection is likely to have psychological effects leading to isolation, maladjusted behaviour, etc. These children have to be provided the most appropriate environment for overcoming difficulties. Though educators at present confine to observable cognitive or sensory disabilities, there are many children who experience emotional problems. It is believed that the society and life systems can also lead to depressions resulting in mental illness.

Methods of Identifying Children with Disabilities

Early identification and intervention are imperative to address many problems of children with disabilities before they become complicated. Therefore, teachers and students must be oriented to the methods of identifying children with disabilities. Some of the following methods may be adopted in this connection:

(a) **Primary Health Centres (PHCs):** The PHC is normally the first contact point for the parents of children with disabilities in rural areas. The doctors of the PHCs need to provide guidance to them regarding facilities for education and rehabilitation of the child. The orientation programme on "Disability Management", being organised by the RCI for the PHC doctors in the country has revealed that doctors are able to refer thousands of persons with disabilities to various education and rehabilitation programmes. Therefore, PHCs are good sources for identifying children with disabilities. As a matter of orientation, teachers and children from schools can visit nearby primary schools to see how children with disabilities come into contact with these PHCs.

(b) **Hospitals:** Established hospitals can provide reliable information regarding the number of disabled children, the incidence and the prevalence of various kinds of disabilities in the particular locality. The general health camps organised by hospitals and other voluntary organisations can also provide necessary information on disabilities.

(c) **Population centers:** The statistics available from population centres may serve as the base for making door-to-door survey to find out the actual number of disabled children for placement in schools.

(d) **Voluntary organisations:** Statistical data regarding the disabled population and expertise for implementation of special education programmes may also be available from voluntary organisations which are involved in the services for persons with disabilities.

(e) **Through school teachers:** Teachers who work in rural areas have more access to the community and they can obtain reliable information from parents, Parents' Association and Parent-Teacher Association regarding the presence of children with disabilities in the community.

(f) **Through school children:** The school teachers may ask non-disabled children of the school to bring information about the children who behave differently while seeing, who fumble over the objects, cannot hear, cannot follow specific directions, etc. On the basis of the information brought by school children, the teacher can pursue the matter for locating disabled children for medical care and placement in school.

(g) **Through village functionaries:** The village head, village administrative officer, village workers, Integrated Child Development Services (ICDS) workers and village nurses can help in the identification of disabled children for placement in schools.

(h) **Census data:** The statistics used at present are the projections from the National Sample Survey Organisation (NSSO) J 99 J. These are only projections and the actual data are yet to be available. The Census 2001 has made an earnest attempt to detect persons with disabilities. When the Census report is available, the information on disability, right from national to block levels, may be clear.

The identification techniques discussed in this section are not exhaustive. Local specific techniques may be designed and used for identification of children with disabilities.

It is evident that definitions of disabilities have a large impact on the nature of services too. Clear definitions help in the effective identification process. Therefore, it is essential for teachers to know about various categories of disabilities. Though they cannot do clinical assessment, functional assessment procedures can be used by them to identify the children, who can be clearly assessed by doctors and specialists for clinical assessment and for proper educational placement.

What Causes Disability?

Disability occurs mainly on account of two reasons. First is the natural disability and second is the artificial or man-made disability. Natural disability means certain persons are disabled by birth. Such persons are born with some physical and mental disorder which are sometime curable some time not. If the disorders are incurable then the persons born with physical or mental disorders have to live rest of the life with the same. Many a time these disabled are 'differently able' by the grace of God, i.e. when God impairs the one faculty of the human being he compensates it by opening the other faculty of human personality. This has existed since the beginnings of humanity and Governments world over have been doing something about it.

The other category of disabled are those which are man-made i.e. disability that occurs on account of accident, war, insurgency, terrorism or militancy and other such activities of human being itself. It is this second category of man-made disability of which the people of the different states of Northeastern India are the worst victim.

The entire population of northeast has been exposed to this man-made disability on account of insurgency and counter-insurgency. Consequently, today it has become a glaring problem of human rights violation on account of the negligence of State and militancy of insurgents or the so-called self-proclaimed freedom fighters. The innocent civilians are the worst victim of this ongoing insurgency and counter-insurgency operations in northeast. Therefore, it has emerged in the form of a deep-rooted social crisis that has a great bearing upon the peace and stability of the region. However, everything is justified on the name of collateral damage, much to the chagrin of the innocent victim of the entire episode.

Disability in Northeast

According to census 2001, in context to the North East states, Meghalaya has the smallest number of disabled persons at 1.24 per cent of its total population with Nagaland coming second at 1.33 per cent. Mizoram is the third state with the smallest population of disabled persons. 1.8 per cent of the state's population had been declared disabled as per government 10 of India guidelines where sight, hearing, speech, movement and mental disabilities were taken into account.

A Person with Disabilities (PWD) in Nagaland is hardly aware about the legislations which are meant for safeguarding him and the institutional mechanism for rehabilitating such persons is non existent in rural areas of the state. A participatory study to understand issues, situation, concerns, needs and aspirations of PWDs in Nagaland found that none of the participants in different villages are aware of the Persons with Disabilities Act, 1995 and none of the persons in the state possesses disability identity cards.

HUMAN RIGHTS APPROACH TO DISABILITY

Constitution of India (1950) Fundamental Rights (Part III) ensures Right to Equality.

Article 14. Equality before law—The State shall not deny any person equality before the law or the equal protection of the laws within the Indian territory.

Article 15. Prohibition of discrimination on grounds of religion, race, caste, sex or place of birth.

(1) The State shall not discriminate against any citizen on grounds only of religion, race, caste, sex, place of birth or any of them.

(2) No citizen shall on grounds only of religion, race, caste, sex, place of birth or any of them, be subject to any disability, liability, restriction or condition with regard to—

  (a) access to shops, public restaurants, hotels and places of public entertainment; or

  (b) the use of wells, tanks, bathing ghats, roads and places of public resort maintained wholly or partly out of State funds.

Universal Declaration of Human Rights (1948)

Article 1 speaks, "All human beings are born free and equal in dignity and rights. They are endowed with reason and conscience and should act towards one another in a spirit of brotherhood."

Article 2 speaks, "Everyone is entitled to all the rights and freedoms set forth in this Declaration, without distinction of any kind, such as race, colour, sex, language, religion, political or other opinion, national or social origin, property, birth or other status. Furthermore, jurisdictional or international status of the country or territory to which a person belongs, whether it be independent, trust, non/self-government or under nay other limitation of sovereignty." Article 3 speaks, "Everyone has the right to life, liberty and security of person."

So investment on education of children with disabilities must be treated as an investment on human capital. This outlook requires a solid human rights approach to disability issues. This approach calls for the treatment of disabled persons as individuals rather than those with extreme qualities.

Human rights approach always lays importance on the child and not on his/her disability. It does not give opportunity for stereotypes. Disability has impact in a variety of ways on education, physical independence, and emotional stability, intellectual and social development of a person. Non-disabled persons tend to generalise the qualities of persons with disabilities due to their limited exposure to them. Their opinion regarding the life of disabled people is mostly stereotyped. Common stereo-type attitudes are:

- "loss of one sense sharpens the other senses"
- "disabled people have more concentration"
- "disabled people have God-given abilities", etc.

This stereotype attitude is directly related to family acceptance or rejection of a disabled person, and, therefore, certainly contributes to discrimination. Moreover, stereotype attitudes force exclusion of persons with disabilities from the society by focusing on their disability conditions. Therefore, stereotypes have to be avoided at all times. Young non-disabled children must be taught that disabled children are children first and disabled next, so that they can appreciate the individuality.

Basic Principles of Human Rights Approach to Education

The goals of Education For All (EFA) in the case of disabled persons can be achieved only when the general education system is geared to meet the educational needs of these children with minimal or no assistance from special teachers. By treating education as the right of the disabled child, the society will be able to see the 'ability of children' rather than harping on their 'disability'. The human rights approach does not label children on the basis of disabilities. The basic principles of human rights approach to education embrace the following:

(a) The human rights approach in education recognizes the fact that every child is special in one way or the other.

The teacher with such an approach realizes that each child has learning ability at different levels. Though classroom instruction, in general, is made uniform irrespective of the intellectual abilities of the children, a good teacher pays attention to the individual capabilities of the children. In such a classroom, the inclusion of all children takes place and they are not categorized on the basis of colour, creed, intellect, disability, etc.

(b) A teacher with human rights approach understands and capitalizes the collective strength of the classroom.
He/she will never hesitate to take help from the students. Rather he/she would use the abilities of the students for constructive purposes. Such a teacher realizes that students – both disabled and non-disabled can also contribute to problem-solving situations in the classroom.

(c) A teacher who believes in human rights approach facilitates peer-to-peer learning.
As this type of learning is non-threatening in nature, the teacher is expected to promote peer group learning as a vehicle to overcome the inhibitions of the students and would gradually make the entire classroom non-threatening. A properly guided peer-group learning activity would make learning faster too. In addition to the pace, the teacher-guided student activity can also make the students responsible for a healthy classroom climate. In such a setting, a child with disability will not experience discrimination.

(d) In an effective classroom, the teacher makes optimum utilisation of the available teaching aids and assistive devices Instead of demanding more and more teaching aids, a creative teacher makes use of the environment itself to develop appropriate concepts. Instead of insisting too much on theoretical learning, the teacher will encourage learning by doing and interactive learning approaches to make optimum use of the teaching aids as well as the environment for effective learning. When the teacher encourages learning by doing, disabled children who require concrete experiences are benefited much.

(e) A good teacher is always conscious of the fact that the students are human beings and not learning machines.
This approach makes the teacher to set realistic goals for the students. Often, the ordinary teacher thinks that his/her subject is the only important subject and loads the students with a lot of homework and assignments. Likewise, other teachers, too, do the same thing and as a result, the student becomes a frustrated human being, not able to complete the home work. This feeling of failure lowers the self-esteem of the child. Teachers should always realize the fact that the students have their limits and, therefore, set learning objectives and provide work which are realistic. As children with disabilities require appropriate curricular adaptations, treating them as individuals facilitates better learning.

(f) A good teacher will adopt multi-sensory approach in learning Learning should be experiential to the students and hence, an effective teacher will make the classroom itself a conducive place for learning. He/she will motivate each and every student of the class to involve in active learning and will be flexible so that children feel free in the classroom. He/she will identify the learning preference—visual, auditory or tactile of the students and facilitate learning through small groups. Even the physical structure of the 82 classroom may be changed by the teacher to ensure effective learning. This multi-sensory approach is not only useful for children with disabilities but for other children too who experience learning problems.

(g) An effective teacher supervises the learning activities of the students regularly.
He/she will try not to find fault with the work of the students but help in rectifying their mistakes through constructive criticism. This positive approach provides better learning environment to children with disabilities.
Human rights approach lays importance to the individual and respecting his/her potentiality in the learning process. 'Recognizing the potential of the individual' is what a child with disability requires in an effective learning environment.

Therefore, adopting human rights approach in the classroom ensures effective teaching and hence better quality of education.

In text materials, too, persons with disabilities should not be projected as fallen souls. Their image should be correctly portrayed in textbooks and media so that the students and public develop positive image about persons with disabilities.

AWARENESS OF ASSISTIVE DEVICES

Training in the use of assistive devices is one of the important parameters of success in the education of children with disabilities. But only provision of these devices would not suffice. The children must be given adequate training to use them. Though these devices are usually taught by specialist teachers, general teachers are also encountering situations to teach these skills, where special teachers are not available. Short-term training in the use of these devices helps the regular teachers to help children with disabilities effectively. Though some equipments are pertinent to specific disability groups, most of the teaching devices can be used in the general classrooms too. Therefore, familiarity with these devices would help the classroom teachers to adopt multi-sensory approaches in teaching. General teachers should realise that there are some areas of learning, particularly the devices, which are peculiar to disability categories. The skills peculiar to disability categories are called 'plus curricular skills'.

Curriculum is the totality of experience attained by the student in the classroom, playground, laboratory, etc. Curriculum meant for non-disabled children should be followed in the education of disabled children without major omissions. In case of MR children, age appropriate need-based functional activities (skills) should be the operational curriculum. Research studies indicate that 80-85 per cent of the general curriculum could be duplicated for disabled children. The rest can also be provided through modified and substituted experiences.

In order to perform well in curricular aspects, disabled children should learn 'plus curricular' activities, as the correlation between general and 'plus curricular' activities is positive and high. The efficiency in 'plus curricular' activities must be emphasized for disabled children and use of devices is one of the important 'plus curricular activities'.

TEACHING METHODS

A good method of teaching is based on multi-sensory approach, whether teaching disabled or non-disabled children. While teaching, the teacher should bear in mind that children with disabilities have reduction in the range and variety of some learning experiences due to their disabilities. However, they should also have the conviction that such reduced experiences can be compensated through effective methods of teaching. In order to facilitate effective teaching learning process, curricular adaptations are imperative. These are important for developing proper conceptual learning too by children with disabilities.

Curricular Adaptations

As inclusive education is one of the most viable options to increase educational opportunities for persons with disabilities, a thorough curricular adaptation is needed for creating better learning environment. As far as possible, the curriculum need not be changed for disabled children since it would work as a criterion for segregation. Adaptations in terms of methods of presentation, display, content, etc., may be necessary to enhance the learning experiences of these children. This approach not only helps children with disabilities, but also helps the teacher to assist children who have learning problems.

The National Institute of Open Schooling has completed a major exercise of adapting secondary education curriculum for the benefit of blind children and such an exercise can be undertaken for other categories of disabilities, wherever necessary. This would improve secondary educational opportunities for all disabled children. Curricular adaptations are mostly suggested for visually impaired children who need non-visual experiences in adaptation of learning materials for the use of children with disabilities.

It is vital to see to what extent the information provided is creating a near normal experience to them. Therefore, adaptation work should be done carefully taking into account the learning style as well as the capacity of the disabled child. In a text material, it is vital to break them into different sub-units and analyse each and every sub-unit and classify the items into visual and non-visual oriented. Further to this analysis, it is essential to indicate at what cognitive level the learning tasks fall so that the teacher can design appropriate strategies for the learning of the child. The cognitive tasks may be categorised as knowledge, understanding, application, analysis, synthesis and evaluation tasks.

The curricular adaptations help children with mental retardation too who require individualised attention. As deaf children have limited communication abilities, the adaptations help them in understanding the content effectively. Therefore, curricular adaptations are most appropriate for effective learning by all types of disabled children.

Concept Development

Concept development is fundamental in the education of children with disabilities, particularly for those who are cognitively impaired such as mentally retarded children; and sensorily impaired such as visually impaired children and hearing impaired children. Loss of one sense of the child adversely affects the concept development of these children. Though specific concept development areas are applicable for specific types of children with disabilities, some concept development areas are general. They include body awareness, object and intuition characteristics, time and distance awareness, spatial awareness, measurements, orientation of environment, etc. These have to be consciously developed in the child. The following are some sample items/concepts pertaining to Concept Development.

- **Body awareness:** Show your left hand, show your stomach, move the head up, spread the feet apart, etc.
- **Object/situation characteristics:** Discrimination of long and short (objects given), hard and soft, identifying colour of objects and characteristics (e.g., leaf and green colour) identifying softness of sound, etc.

- **Time and distance awareness:** Which month comes after July, the sun rises approximately at 6.00 a.m./10.00 a.m./2.00 p.m./ 9.00 p.m.; how many meters form a kilometre, etc.
- **Spatial awareness:** Turn about, walk in zigzag position, sound localisation, direction, etc.
- **Skills oriented (action) concepts:** Crawling, kicking the ball, pulling the chair, rotating the head, etc.
- **Measurements:** More and less (objects given), how many twos in ten, place value of numbers, etc.
- **Orientation of environment:** What do you mean by river, post office, plant, cloud, etc.

As most of these concepts grow naturally in a non-disabled child, a disabled child living in the mainstreaming environment will be able to acquire these concepts in a natural way.

Therefore, inclusive education setting is more conducive for the concept development of children with disabilities. Even in the special schools, the children can be provided ample opportunities to develop their concept development skills.

Teaching Subject Areas

In education of children with disabilities, it is often believed that children require different methodologies for learning purposes. In fact, this attitude, which prevailed for decades contributed to exclusive concepts like special schools. Though it is true in some cases, most of the subject areas do not require any substantial changes. Children with disabilities do not require a separate method of teaching. A good teacher is expected to use approaches which would enable all children to study effectively, irrespective of their disability. Therefore, the inclusive education setting emphasises on curricular adaptations rather than prescribing a new curriculum.

Some methods of teaching which can be useful for children with disabilities are listed as follows:

Play-way method

In this method, the child is not kept in the classroom as a learner.

The child is introduced the lesson through a number of play activities and in the process of such play, the teacher introduces specific concepts. Children who are learning through play-way method experience a sense of discovery.

Providing concrete experiences

Children learn in three developmental stages. First, they need concrete experiences involving three dimensional objects, etc. Secondly, they can learn through pictorial ideas, and thirdly they develop abstraction. As far as children with disabilities are concerned, providing concrete learning experiences becomes pertinent. A strong foundation developed through concrete experiences will help them to understand the higher order experiences, including those of abstraction without much difficulty.

Facilitating learning by involving children with disabilities in groups

Cooperative learning approach is considered to be an effective teaching-learning process in the classroom, especially when the class has children of different abilities. In a class consisting of children with disabilities, group learning can be planned by involving a child with disability in a group consisting of non-disabled children. This kind of activity not only develops the academic skills but also influences social integration of the child.

Teacher assisted peer-group learning

Peer group learning is considered to contribute to effective learning in the case of non-disabled children and it is not less so in the case of disabled children. For adopting peer-group learning, a lot of preparation on the part of the teacher is needed. Activities for peer group learning, strategies for intervention, etc., are to be thoroughly planned by the teacher. A teacher in this process can become the facilitator of information sharing and see that the children (including disabled children) study in a harmonious way.

Teaching in a step-by-step way

Due to the loss of a specific faculty, children with disabilities are bound to lose the sequence of learning experiences. They often experience mediated learning and as a result, they need well-defined learning strategies. Teaching in a step-by-step sequence becomes vital for children with disabilities. Though this type of incremental approach is helping all children, children with disabilities are very much benefited by this. They are able to overcome the loss of learning experiences which are forced by the absence of the senses, when teaching is done in a step-by-step way.

Modifying method of teaching to suit the individual learning styles of disabled children

The teacher should ascertain whether the child is a visual learner or an auditory learner or a tactile learner for designing proper instructional strategies. Though classification of this kind is imperative in the general classroom too, its application with children with disabilities is of paramount importance because these children exhibit different skills at different levels.

Criterion based teaching as well as evaluation techniques

Usually, evaluation in a regular classroom is norm-based. The teacher makes an evaluation of the child on the basis of quantitative scores. However, this type of evaluation may not be proper for all activities in the case of children with disabilities. Since disabled children have to learn curricular as well as 'plus curricular' activities, mastery of the child over certain skills is more important than comparing the child with another child. Therefore, criterion-based evaluation is appropriate, which will help to see the position of the child at various points of time. In criterion-based evaluation, there is no pressure of comparative performance and, therefore, the child can learn in a natural way.

Learning through field-trips and hands-on experience

Since children with disability experience reduction in the range and variety of experiences in many aspects, they have to be compensated by alternative modes of information. Field trips are such alternative experiences which mostly contribute to proper concept development of these children.

Use of supplementary teaching aids and appliances for developing appropriate concepts

As already indicated, concept development is vital for the disabled child to understand academic as well as non-academic areas. Sometimes, a concept taught by the teacher using the normal mode of information may not be appropriate for the child with disability to understand. Therefore, it is essential to use additional teaching aids which may provide the needed concept development in the child. The supplementary teaching aids should not be considered as additional burden. In fact, these are to be treated as essential for providing the substituted learning experiences to children with disabilities.

Individualised Education Programmes

For specific categories, such as mentally retarded children, their needs and abilities must be assessed and appropriate instructional strategies must be designed and addressed based on their strengths and needs. It includes medical, social and psycho-educational interventions.

When the above aspects are addressed by the regular classroom teacher, teaching of any subject would become easier for the disabled child to understand. Therefore, practice-oriented teaching approach would enhance the learning efficiencies of disabled children.

CLASSROOM ACTIVITIES TOWARDS REDUCING DISCRIMINATION

Learning Process

Learning is change of behaviour and a positive change in the behaviour occurs when the learning environment is non-threatening. In such a conducive learning environment, learning becomes effective and the teacher and the taught mutually facilitate learning experiences. An effective teacher never assumes the role of just a giver of information and he/she will not treat the taught as the mere recipient of knowledge. Therefore, an effective learning environment reinforces good practices of the classroom. In an effective classroom, the teacher would address the needs of all children, irrespective of their abilities or disabilities.

Normally, young children do not have the tendency to discriminate. They may be curious to know about disability conditions but do not have the tendency to isolate children on the basis of sex, caste, religion, disability, etc. As the child grows, prejudices also grow and as a result, discrimination takes place. In order to reduce the discriminatory approaches, positive orientation can be given to non-disabled children. As children have a tendency to extend over-help to children with disabilities, they have to be informed to be natural and should not over-do when they help children with disabilities. This type of orientation is necessary when the child with disability is integrated in the general classrooms.

Cooperative Learning Approach

Cooperative learning approach addresses these issues and when it is followed, it produces better results. Cooperative learning approach adopts three fundamental hypotheses:

(i) Every child is a special child.
(ii) A child with disability is MORE LIKE than UNLIKE.
(iii) A teacher becomes a facilitator of learning.

When these principles are practised in letter and spirit, the inclusion of children with disabilities would become natural. In applying cooperative learning approach, a teacher may like to involve student participation in the learning process. Soon after teaching a lesson, the students may be asked to work in small groups on specific themes. The group formation may be based on the alphabetical order, height of the students, etc., and the teacher should ensure that there is a disabled child in each small group. On any account, the "teacher should not leave group formation to the discretion of the students. The thematic discussion should be monitored by the teacher. Once the thematic discussion is over, the teacher should facilitate inter-group discussion by bringing one student from each group together to form a new group. In the inter-group discussion, each student, including the disabled student, will be assuming the role of a teacher; when his/her turn comes, he/she explains to other students what was discussed in the thematic groups, etc. This activity improves the communication skills of the learners and every student in the class is expected to speak. As all students in the class should take part in the learning activity, all of them should receive equal attention of the teacher. After a thorough inter-group discussion, the teacher should bring the class back and put questions to examine the understanding of the students. Based on the understanding level, the teacher can recapitulate the learning points and provide further assignments for enrichment. As evident from the description, cooperative learning is not only a technique to facilitate effective inclusion of children with disabilities, but is an effective teaching methodology too to help all children.

Cooperative learning is a carefully organized peer-to-peer learning activity in which the characteristics of group dynamics are thoroughly dealt with. This carefully planned learning activity through peer-group interaction is likely to enhance the learning experiences of disabled and non-disabled students.

SIMULATION EXERCISES ABOUT DISABILITIES

Simulation exercises about disability may be fun but they have profound educational values. In order to simulate disability conditions, non-disabled children in the general classrooms may be blindfolded for some time, their ears plugged for some time, and they can also be asked to walk using one leg, write without the help of thumb, etc., to experience disability conditions of different nature. Often, non-disabled children find simulating exercises as fun and, therefore, like to have them. At the same time, they can also understand how children with disabilities live and learn. This type of simulating exercises would improve the concern of non-disabled children towards their disabled classmates. These activities also facilitate better inclusion of disabled children in the classroom. Teachers can also experience these simulating activities to understand various conditions of disabilities.

Learning 'Plus Curricular Activities' by Non-Disabled Children

'Plus curricular activities' are those which are peculiar to specific disability conditions and they are expected to be mastered by children with disabilities for their effective inclusion. However, orientation of these to non-disabled children would facilitate better inclusion for children with disabilities. For example, the braille dots can be taught to sighted children. Similarly, a few basic signs used by deaf children can be taught to hearing children so that they can communicate with deaf children. Disabled children appreciate non-disabled children studying these skills as they bring them closer to the mainstream.

Reader and Scribe Services

Due to disability conditions, some of them need assistance during examination time. For example, a blind child may not be able to read volumes of Braille books at the time of examination. Moreover, many textbooks are also not available in braille and, therefore, a blind child needs a reader. A child with cerebral palsy and a child with mild mental retardation may also be benefited by reader services. At the examination time, a blind child and a child with cerebral palsy may require a scribe to write the answers. In inclusive setting, many such examinations, class tests, term-end examinations, etc., are conducted and, therefore, a number of non-disabled children from the same class, or from higher classes may be involved to assist children with disabilities. Similarly, non-disabled children who have picked up some signs may be used to interpret the language of deaf children to others.

The above activities provide ample opportunities for disabled children and non-disabled children to interact effectively in the' learning process. The activities listed, however, are not exhaustive. Other activities such as drama, skit, role play, etc., involving disabled and non-disabled persons may also provide opportunities for effective inclusion of disabled children in the mainstream society, thereby reducing discrimination.

School Based Activities to Develop Non-Discrimination

The following activities may be practised by students and teachers in the general school environment to exercise the value of non-discrimination.

1. Awareness programmes on disability management may be

organized for non-disabled children in general schools to expose them to the various conditions of disability.

2. Persons with disabilities may be invited to address non-disabled children on how disabled persons manage day-to-day activities. The interaction between disabled and non-disabled persons might help teachers in breaking barriers in respect of attitude.
3. Lessons projecting the right image about persons with disabilities may be included in the curriculum of schools right from the beginning. Similarly, pictures portraying the right image of persons with disabilities should also be included at the primary level itself.
4. Simulating exercises such as blind-folding of sighted children to experience the conditions of persons with blindness, plugging the ears for sometime to simulate the conditions of deaf persons, etc., may be useful for non-disabled persons to understand the conditions of persons with disabilities.
5. Adapted physical education activities may be encouraged in general schools wherein persons with disabilities may be encouraged to play with non-disabled children.
6. Non-disabled children can be taken to schools for persons with disabilities and other service centres to see the activities of persons with disabilities.
7. The concept of abilympics, which provide opportunities for persons with disabilities to demonstrate their vocational skills in various trades, is becoming popular now.

   These activities may be organized in various parts of the country to enable non-disabled persons to see the activities of persons with disabilities.
8. Summer camps may be organized by schools to take persons with disabilities along with non-disabled children to interact socially to develop positive awareness about disability issues.
9. Parents of disabled children may be brought to address teachers in general schools and also in Parent-Teacher Associations to highlight the abilities of persons with disabilities.

10. The regular teacher may involve disabled children in a number of group activities with non-disabled children both inside and outside the classroom. For example, the disabled child may be involved in a group performing scientific experiment to note down the descriptions given by other persons, etc.
11. The teacher may be advised to include disabled children in field trips and encourage the peers to care for them to explain about the places visited.
12. The teachers may be advised to include children with disabilities in extra-curricular activities such as drama, dance etc.
13. The senior students may be motivated to act as scribe for visually impaired children.
14. Peer tutoring involving disabled and non-disabled children may be encouraged.
15. Opportunity may be given to disabled children to develop their leadership qualities by asking them to organize various activities.
16. In the hostel settings, the disabled students should not be provided a separate room and a separate place for dining. They should be given an opportunity to mingle with non-disabled children.
17. Teaching aids for any lesson should be prepared keeping in mind the difficulties of disabled children.
18. Refresher courses should be conducted for the teachers about the current trends and issues in the field of rehabilitation.
19. Architectural barriers should be removed while constructing school buildings.
20. Lives of successful disabled persons should be taught to students.
21. Students may be asked to collect success stories of disabled persons from magazines.
22. Teachers should ask every student whether any of their close relatives are disabled. They should be asked to share their experiences with other children.

23. Students should be encouraged to frequently visit, talk and write to their grand parents who may suffer from degenerative disorders due to old age.

PSYCHO-SOCIAL IMPLICATIONS OF DISABILITIES

Disability conditions have many implications for the life of the affected individual. They have direct and indirect impact on their psychological development as well as in the sociological front.

Three types of implications are normally caused because of disability.

- Firstly, the disability itself causes emotional upset in the individual.
- Secondly, it is important to know in what aspects it affects the personality traits of the individual. Psychological aspects such as self-concept, self-esteem, perception, and the sub-needs such as intimacy, success, autonomy and self-expression, self-worthiness, etc. are affected as a result of disability conditions.
- Thirdly, it is necessary to know to what extent the psychological implications have impact on the sociological factors such as family acceptance, social integration, etc. The development in psycho-social adjustment of the person with disability, emotional maturity and dependability will make him eligible for acceptance by the society for meaningful living.

Really speaking, psycho-social development of persons with disabilities is not affected so much by the disability, but it is disrupted by the emotional overtones of the disability. It is now a well-known fact that children tend to achieve as much, and only as much, as their parents aspire them to achieve. Once parents stop treating the child as a developing individual, once they refuse to accept his capabilities and limitations, both, in a realistic manner, his/her self-concept is bound to be severely affected. Over-protection robs him/her of his/her independence; neglect turns him/her to undesirable behaviours. Either way, it is the suffering child whose handicap multiplies. The same is true with the society. Society should not exercise stereotype attitudes towards disabilities, which cause either exclusion or too much care. For better psycho-social development, the society should treat the persons with disability as individuals.

Effects of Disability on Personality

Personality is treated as the total quality of the individual's behaviour as it is revealed in his/her thought, action, expression and attitude. Among these, the attitude forms the base for all other components and undoubtedly contributes to the development of the self-esteem of the individual. In the case of disabled persons, their attitudes toward the world and vice-versa play an important role in the making up of the self. Disability conditions have many effects on the development of the individual. As abilities such as understanding the environment, communication, reasoning, access, etc, have direct influence on the personality, a person with disability would certainly experience limitations in these areas, which may cause psychological effect on the personality.

Compensatory activities to combat these effects would contribute to better personality development in the individual. Early intervention and remedial activities alone contribute to a balanced personality development in persons with disabilities.

Role of Persons with Disabilities

In the personality development, the person with disability has a vital role. The individual, though upset by the disability condition, should cultivate the mind to live with disability and overcome the difficulties. Though it is easier said than experienced, the determination of the disabled individual to live and face the challenges of the world has a tremendous impact on the positive development of the individual. As the society at large has a tendency to provide importance to the abilities of the individual, a person with disability should also develop his/her ability to easily get into the mainstream. Accepting the disability as it is and moving forward from there with constructive thinking would contribute to a balanced personality development of the individual.

The personality development of the disabled individual is not only influenced by the external forces but by the determination of the individual too.

Role of Peer Groups

Peer group influence is substantial in the making of individuals, whether it is in the childhood, adulthood or in old age. A disabled individual should have better interaction with other disabled persons and also non-disabled persons of the same age group. Experiences have revealed that disabled children, integrated with the mainstream programmes, tend to accept the disability condition and move forward for constructive life. Therefore, disabled persons should be mainstreamed as early as possible to experience the positive effects of personality development on the individual with disability.

Role of Parents

Parents are the most important people in the life of the non-disabled child as also that of the children with disability. The habilitation and/or rehabilitation of the disabled child should, in fact, start from the family. The parents are generally ignorant about implications of disability on the personality development of the child. In most of the places, parents also like to render maximum assistance to disabled children. But their unawareness of the right methodology in the treatment of such children keeps them away from providing possible assistance. This is the time for the schools and organizations working for persons with disabilities to offer guidance and counselling programmes to the families of these children. It is, therefore, very evident that the parents of these children should be involved in planning the educational programmes for them.

It is essential, however, to make sure that parents understand the following aspects:

1. Reasons for disability condition in the child and its implications for the present.
2. The effect of the disability condition of the child on his/her concept development.
3. Ways of helping the child at home to develop his/her skills.
4. Understanding the skill areas and limitations of the child.
5. The need for praise and encouragement for social and emotional development.

6. Need for cooperation with the Early Childhood Care and Education (ECCE) programmes and the teachers for improving skills of the child.

In short, parents need to playa pro-active role in the personality development of the child with disabilities.

Overall Value Development

In the life of the child with disabilities, education, vocation, family acceptance and social integration become the four vital pillars. Parents, teachers, peer group and the society at large have their respective roles in the overall development of the child. Besides the psychological, sociological and personality development of the child, the value development is also vital. Value development activities not only contribute to effective personality development, but also provide courage to encounter the challenges imposed by disability conditions. As cultivation of the mind is the basic requirement for value development, meditation and yoga activities may also be practised with persons with disabilities.

Role of Teachers

The teachers should help the parents to observe disabled children in the classroom settings and notice the nature of training he/she needs in language, cognitive, motor, emotional and social developments. The teachers should encourage parents to ask questions and clarify doubts. Moreover, the parents should be oriented by the teachers to identify the areas where the child needs maximum assistance. In general, close collaboration of the teachers and parents of disabled children could make a tremendous impact on the overall development of the child. Teachers should also assume advocacy roles. Their knowledge on special assistance, sources and agencies which are locally or proximally available will equip them to play an effective role as referral teachers. They need not be resource persons, but must have information on supportive services. They should be aware of the legal right protection, schemes and benefits for disabled persons.

Often, teachers are looked upon by parents and disabled children as the major source for guidance. As teachers are trained to handle children with disabilities in the professional way, their influence on the personality development of the child is undisputable. They should act as mentors for children with disabilities and their parents. If possible, making visits to the families of children with disabilities and interacting with the child, their parents and siblings may have a positive influence on the personal\ty development of the child. Therefore, teachers should continue to playa facilitative role in special education.

IMPLICATIONS FOR TEACHER EDUCATION

National Policy on Education (1986/1992)

A significant exhortation in the National Policy on Education (NPE) 1986 with modifications undertaken in 1992 incorporates the basic spirit of Article 51A and reads thus: "The National System of Education will be based on a national curricular framework which contains a common core along with other components that are flexible. The common core will include the history of India's freedom movement, the Constitutional obligations and other content essential to nurture national identity. These elements will cut across subject areas and will be designed to promote values such as India's common cultural heritage; egalitarianism, democracy and secularism; equality of the sexes; protection of the environment; removal of social barriers; observance of the small family norm, and inculcation of the scientific temper. All educational programmes will be carried on in strict conformity with secular values." This policy statement reinforces the concern for a total curriculum renovation.

Reorienting Teacher Education Programmes

It is not enough that the teachers are made aware of the Constitutional provisions about equality and the need for non-discrimination; it will also require educating them in communicating these ideas to the students and impressing on them the need to abide by the dictums of the same. For a serious business of education in Constitutional concerns at the school level, teachers of all subjects at all levels have to be oriented and trained. Accordingly, the curricular coverage of these concepts has to be deliberate and pre-designed. It will be necessary to develop a blueprint indicating reflection of various concerns in different units and topics of the course papers in teacher education curricula. Preparation of teachers, through well-designed teacher education programmes, would actually play very significant role in ensuring understanding and internalizing of these concepts in our schools, teacher education institutions and communities.

Towards reorienting teacher education which is the most crucial input in operationalizing the ideas mentioned in the preceding chapters, a few suggestions are given below only as guidelines, hoping that the teacher educators will be able to apply their own minds to designing approaches to the implementation of the ideas in various innovative ways.

Conclusion

Disabled children are human beings like others. They should not be discriminated because they are different. They are part of the contributing citizens of the society. Teachers should avoid discriminatory measures and include children with disabilities in the mainstream of education. In short, a general school should have the following pro-active objectives regarding education of children with disabilities to enforce the need for non-discrimination.

1. The purpose of education is to provide equal educational opportunities as well as experiences to children with disabilities.
2. Schools should provide least restrictive environment to persons with disabilities in order to maximise their social experiences.
3. Schools should start activities to overcome stereotype attitudes towards disability by demonstrating that disabled children are children first and disabled next.
4. Schools should invest on the education of children with disabilities to make them contributing citizens of the nation.

In summary, non-discriminatory practices start with the formation of the right attitude. In this process, teachers can playa crucial role in developing such attitudes among non-disabled children to practice non-discrimination based on caste, gender, religion and disability.

REFERENCES

1. Dev, A., Dev, I.A. and Das, S. (1996): Human Rights: A Source Book. Delhi: NCERT.
2. Diane Tillman (2000): Living Values Activities for Young Adults. Delhi: Sterling Publishers.
3. Hassija, J.C. (1983): Eternal Drama of Soul, Matter and God. Delhi: Brahma Kumaris,
4. Hassija, J.C. (1997): Human Rights Education. Mount Abu: Brahma Kumaris.
5. Krippner, S. and Rubin, D. (Ed) (1975): The Energy of Consciousness. New York: Garden and Breach.
6. Peck, R.F. and Havighurst, R.J. (1960): The Psychology of Character Development. New York: Willey.
7. Rama Jois, M. (1997): Human Rights and Indian Values. Delhi: NCTE.
8. Sahoo, Jayadeba (1995). Human Rights, Indian Cultural Heritage, Values and Education: A Critical Analysis. University News. 43 (50):85-99.
9. Shanmugam, T.E. (1987). Community Psychology. Madras: Utsav Shanmugam.

Web Sites: http// www.livingvalues.net ; www.bkwsu.com

PART III

DISABILITY AND HUMAN RIGHTS

8

Disabled in India: Imperatives for Rethinking Legal and Policy Interventions

Alok Kumar Gupta and Geetanjali Sharma

Introduction

Salil Chaturvedi who was rendered crippled after a fateful accident at the age of 16, became the first differently abled Indian to have sailed from Mumbai to Goa. He bravely claims that "*Though initially my disability made me a bit of an outsider yet today, this has made me insightful and sensitive to the synergies of the universe. It has also, to a large extent, shaped my decisions, goal and philosophy of life.*"[1] But sadly this is not the best example to describe the state of differently abled in India.

The present population of India is 102 crores and approximately 5-6 per cent of the total population which amounts to around 6.12 crores are estimated to be differently abled in one form or the other. According to the World Bank estimates India has some 40 to 80 million persons with disability and at least one in every 12 household has a member with disability. Children with disability are 5 times more likely to be out of school than average.[2] Despite this huge number the policy response as well the legislations which are there in place are not adequate enough to address the problems in terms of need and aspirations of these people.

Most vital is the attitude of people, society and community in general towards a differently-abled person which in turn tends to have a profound impact on the policy decisions. As two Indian authors have put it, "At a profoundly serious and spiritual level, disability represents divine justice".[3] At a more mundane level, people with disabilities are traditionally perceived as somehow inauspicious. Much qualitative research has found considerable social marginalisation of people with disabilities in India, though most also acknowledge that the social status of the PWD's (Person with disability) family has an impact on their potential acceptance in society.

Another vital aspect is the tool of legislation which addresses the needs of the society. Legislation in this regard could be Special, General or a mixture of Special and General. The legislation must cover the following areas of a differently-abled life: Education, Employment, the right to marriage, the right to family/parenthood, Political Laws, Accessibility to the court of law, Right to privacy, Property Rights. It should be ensured that the benefits to a differently abled person must accrue in the form of: Health/Medical care, Rehabilitation, Financial security, Employment, Independent living and Participation in decisions affecting themselves. Thus and emphasis of a national policy must be for the sale of: Prevention, Rehabilitation, Individual Support, Accessibility measures in terms of outdoor facilities, public places, transport, housing etc. and Anti-Discriminatory Laws.

In the light of these factors, the paper aims to trace the debatable issues that have emerged in the course of various disability movements in India. It further attempts to analyze the existing legislations and policy responses and their efficacy in meeting the needs of the people.

Disability Movements: Emerging Issues

1. **Of versus for**: The huge ideological divide between organisations *of* persons with disabilities on one hand, and organisations *for* persons with disabilities on the other, is quite apparent in our country. The advocates of the former

category uphold the view that the leadership, control, and management of disability related organisations must rest with persons with disabilities. They contend that such persons can think, speak, decide, and act for themselves, and that they do not need any mouthpiece albeit they most certainly welcome the support and solidarity of the larger civil society. The opponents of this view feel that the time is not yet ripe for persons with disabilities living in India to organise as they still continue to live in a state of utter disempowerment and disarticulation. This view appears to be driven more by feeling of philanthropy and charity, and perhaps having scant regard for the immense and enormous potential, and capabilities of persons with disabilities.

2. **Cross vs. Uni-disability**: Two categories of organisations on disability rights have emerged over the years. The cross-disability organisations fight for the rights of all persons with disabilities regardless of the nature, extent, or category of disability. The upholders of this category of organisation stress upon the commonality of issues including discrimination, exclusion, and access on an equal basis with others. They assert that persons with disabilities suffer discrimination and exclusion on the basis of long-term physical, mental, intellectual, and sensory impairments. Contrary to this view, there are others who are of the opinion that each category of persons with disabilities have issues specific to the nature, extent, and category of disability which do not often get adequately and equally highlighted through cross-disability organisations hence, the need for Uni-disability organisations.
3. **Community vs. institution**: The seventies and eighties of the last century saw the emergence of the concept of Community Based Rehabilitation (CBR) as opposed to Institution Based Rehabilitation (IBR). This approach envisages, among other things, community ownership of the responsibility and obligation of taking care of the all-round development of persons with disabilities living in a given community. It stresses the need for making available to

persons with disabilities services at their doorstep. The idea is to ensure that persons with disabilities are able to live independently within their own communities. Institution-based rehabilitation, however, envisages training, education, etc, of persons with disabilities in institutional settings where all the facilities expertise pertaining to a given disability are available. The detractors of the CBR approach argue that in developing countries in particular, communities have neither the requisite facilities nor the expertise to appropriately train, educate, and groom a person with disability to lead a life of honour and dignity. In any case, they maintain that expertise, assistive aids and appliances, etc. must come from institutions only.

4. **Special vs. inclusive schools:** There also exist two schools of thought in respect of settings in which education may be imparted to children with disabilities. Those favouring a special school system argue that it is only in special settings that children with disabilities can get quality education, adequate attention and all the required facilities; and that too in an appropriate atmosphere with a level playing field and without feeling excluded in the crowd of non-differently abled children. Such settings ensure that the children with disabilities are able to keep pace with the class unlike in the so-called integrated/inclusive settings. Contrary to the above view, the exponents of integrated/inclusive settings attack the special school system vehemently on the ground that such a system tends to ghettoise children with disabilities. Strongly favouring the idea of working towards creating an inclusive, barrier-free, and rights-based society, they assert that a vast majority of children with disabilities can be accommodated within the regular school settings, and hence, in an inclusive environment, with some adaptations.
5. **Reservation debate:** While a sizeable chunk of people favour the idea of reservations in jobs and other concessions for persons with disabilities, there is a section of people who feel otherwise. People belonging to this latter section contend that since persons with disabilities claim the rights and

privileges of class I citizens, they should not shy away from assuming the responsibilities and obligations that come with such citizenship. However, those who favour such reservation and concessions put forth the view that persons with disabilities are amongst groups which have a long history of marginalisation and exclusion necessitating reservations and concessions etc within the larger framework of affirmative action. They further maintain that such reservation and facilities are being made available to many other disadvantaged and marginalised groups as well.

6. **Jobs identification:** Some people in the disability rights movement favour the idea that persons with disabilities cannot perform all the jobs and that the bureaucrats often are found groping in the dark as to where to place a person with a disability. Section 32 of the Persons with Disability Act 1995 also envisages provision for identification of jobs. It also provides for periodic updation and revision of the list of identified jobs on a regular basis so as to take note of the advancements made in the field of science and technology enabling persons with disabilities to perform greater number of jobs than in the past. Contrary to the above view, there is a section of people that subscribes to the opinion that identification of jobs is redundant, and is pernicious inasmuch as it restricts the scope for persons with disabilities. People favouring this line of thinking, further assert that nobody, whether differently abled or non differently abled is capable of performing all the jobs under the sun. If a person with a disability is incompetent to handle a given job, he anyways stands to be disqualified in the interview itself.
7. **Decision-making mechanism:** The deliberations of the ad-hoc committee on the UN Convention for the Rights of Persons with Disabilities, which later got adopted, witnessed an absorbing battle of wits on the issue of legal capacity of persons with disabilities. While everyone agreed to recognise persons with disabilities as persons before the law on an equal basis with others, and also their legal capacity to act, opinion was divided in respect of persons with certain specific

categories of disabilities, particularly persons with Mental/ Psychosocial disabilities. Some argued that for persons with certain specific categories of disabilities, there should be provision of substituted decision making mechanism since they cannot act on their own. Others, however, felt that for such categories of persons, there should be provision of *supported* decision making mechanism and not for *substituted* decision making mechanism. Supported decision making pre-supposes an inherent capacity in every individual. It also underscored the principle of interdependence amongst human beings. Substituted decision making, on the other hand negates capacity and forecloses all opportunities for a person's capacity to evolve.[4]

Apart from the above mentioned issues, there are certain emerging issues like increasing number of crime rates against differently abled people as well as that of sexual and reproductive rights of the disabled women which are being much debated in the academic circles yet no conclusive policy could be evolved to address them.

Analysis of Existing Legislations

There is no universally agreed definition of disability in our country but, The Persons with Disabilities (Equal Opportunities, Protection of Rights and Full Participation) Act, 1995 (here after The PWD Act) defines disability as one or more of the following: "blindness, low vision, leprosy cured, hearing impairment, locomotor disability, mental retardation and mental illness." To be considered differently abled, a person must suffer from not less than 40 per cent of any disability, as certified by a medical authority. An insight into the existing legislations in our country with respect to the provisions of the UN Convention on Disability highlights the following observations:

1. **PWD Act:** The PWD Act was enacted in 1995, and is known to be one of the best and comprehensive among disability legislation in the countries of the region. However, it suffers from an indistinct terminology and lacks teeth for its full implementation. The definition of this disability

within this Act is highly narrow as compared to Article 1 of the UN Convention which includes all long-term physical, mental, intellectual or sensory impairments which may hinder their full and effective participation in society as disability. Further, the caveat in the PWD Act that reforms should only be undertaken within the limits of a state's economic capacity nullifies the Acts potential for change as Article 4(2) of the Convention clearly says that the maximum possible resources should be utilized for the upliftment of the differently abled. Further, Articles 6 and 7 of the Convention specifically mentions women and children who face greater problems in terms of their disability and states that special provisions need to be made for them. The PWD Act is completely lacking in this respect and needs amendment in order to comply with the Convention. Further, the provisions of access to justice, liberty and security etc. (as espoused in Articles 13 and 14, respectively) do not find much mention in the PWD Act, which deals more with the procedural aspects of disability legislation-with rather elaborate details of the committees to be set up.

2. **The Mental Health Act:** The emphasis of this legislation is on the appointments or qualifications of authorities, admission and discharge of mentally ill from specialized institutions, removal and role of medical officers, magistrates or police officers, liability to meet the cost of maintenance of mentally ill persons, and penalties and punishments, etc. However, there are serious doubts as to the effectiveness of this legislation for ensuring the protection of the person, property and privacy of communication of mentally ill. It leaves sufficient space for the misuse of power by the police, medical officer or magistrate. The percentage of involuntary admissions is often found to be very high and the provisions of Section 19 which permits admission under certain special circumstances by a relative or a friend are being widely abused. The fundamental weakness of the Act is that it perceives institutional care as the only arrangement for the care and protection of persons with mental illness. The

Convention on the other hand aims at restoring the dignity of the differently abled person; it is therefore evident that changes need to be incorporated into this Act to make it more useful to mentally differently abled people.

3. **The RCI Act:** The Rehabilitation Council of India (RCI) came to be established in 1986, followed by an Act to implement its objects in 1992. In essence, the Council and its Act, aims to regulate the quality of training of Rehabilitation Professionals and to maintain a Central Rehabilitation Registration Register of the professionals so trained. However, both the Council and the Act did not find favour the voluntary sector, and a number of problems as highlighted below reflect on the changes that need to be incorporated to make the Act comply with the Convention:
   - Arbitrariness in formulation and implementation.
   - Delay in implementation of the clauses of the Act.
   - Inclusion of the clause of disciplinary action against those who failed to comply with the dictates of the Act.
   - Inadequate definition of the term Rehabilitation professional.
4. **National Trust Act (The National Trust for Welfare of Persons with Autism, Cerebral Palsy, Mental Retardation and Multiple Disabilities Act, 1999):** As certain groups among the differently abled are more vulnerable than others, an enactment for the protection of such persons, their property and well-being was felt necessary. The enactment of the National Trust for Welfare of Persons with Autism, Cerebral Palsy, Mental Retardation and Multiple Disabilities Act, 1999 (Trust Act), was meant to fulfill a common demand of families that seek State provision for their severely differently abled wards. The issue of appointing a guardian under the tenets of this law is governed by the constitution of a local level committee, consisting of an officer of the State, a representative of an NGO and a (any) person with a disability. Throughout the Act, as one weaves through the clauses and sub clauses, there appears to be no involvement of the person with the disability (even notionally). In order

to comply with the spirit and the letter of the Convention, a more comprehensively drafted enactment is needed, which takes into consideration the preferences of the differently abled person, as opposed to merely the relatives or friends.

5. **Child Rights, Education and Disability:** The National Policy on Education was implemented in 1986 to achieve the goal of providing education for all, including the differently abled. Its objective was to integrate the physically and the mentally handicapped with the general community. However, its very wording is faulty, for it envisages *wherever possible* education for the children with motor and other handicaps will be with others Special schools will be provided *as far as possible* for severely handicapped children. When the legislated policy itself is so weakly worded and has no regulatory or enforcement mechanism attached with it, the provisions of the Convention cannot be complied with; unless the resources of the State are diverted into this area of need as per the provisions laid down in the Convention. This is further reflected in the Plan of Action drafted in 1986, which stresses that since the education of handicapped in special schools is very expensive, it will only be for special cases. This neglect to take into account that the special needs of the differently abled often extend beyond the mere basics, and to think that once they have learnt how to read and communicate they can be reintegrated into the mainstream education system is fallacious and is exactly the attitude that the Convention rallies against. The Integrated Education for Differently abled Children, the Bharathi Braille for Visually Impaired Children are all positive steps, which when implemented can help further the cause espoused by the Convention. However, a number of drastic changes are needed to make them relevant in contemporary age.

6. **Disability in the Workplace:** Because the differently abled frequently receive no formal education, their working lives often begin earlier than those of their non-differently abled peers. Furthermore, because they are rarely trained or apprenticed for a specific trade or skill, they are often sent

to work at the most menial jobs, constituting some of the harshest forms of labor. While it is known that many differently abled children are in the workplace, little information on them exists because most find work in informal sectors of society - as house servants, farm workers, in shops or in factories. Because finding and keeping work for individuals with disability is difficult in most societies - (i.e., even in developed countries, the unemployment rate for adults with disability often is above 80 per cent) especially in India, the differently abled children and adolescents have little voice in the workplace and are at risk not only for physical, sexual and verbal abuse, but are also less likely to report such abuse or to quit should they be abused. It becomes increasingly grave and complex in the wake of no social security for the differently abled, and one is faced with abysmal working and labour conditions for people with disabilities; the exact situation that the Convention is trying so vociferously to remove. In order to comply with the convention, therefore, a number of changes to the industrial and labour laws requires to be done, ensuring special protection, privileges and social security for the differently abled.[5]

Policy Responses and Civil Society

Apart from the above mentioned legal regimes to address the issue of the human rights of the Disabled, the government has also taken certain policy decisions or has proposed to take some actions with regards to enhancement of the scope of the rights of the disabled in terms of better accessibility towards resources. The role of media and civil society is equally laudable. Some of the instances to prove the same would be:

- **Easier Identification**: The disability certificate is crucial for a disadvantaged person as it makes him or her eligible to apply for facilities, concessions and benefits under schemes of governments or non-government organisations. In this regard, the Centre recently announced amendments to the Persons with Disabilities (Equal Opportunities, Protection of Rights and Full Participation) Rules, 1996, where the differently-abled now have to appear before only one doctor specialising in the nature of disability instead of going to a Medical Board, which used to be a time consuming process. Also the Primary Health Centre (PHC) doctors have been given the right to issue disability certificate in cases of severe disability, while others with partial disability will still have to go to the District Hospital to get one.[6] But those with complicated disabilities not easily discernible and which need to be assessed scientifically will still have to get the certificate from the district medical boards.[7]

- **Right to Food Security**: Recently Brinda Karat, CPI (M) Polit Bureau member assured a state based organisation working for disabled that the Left Party MPs would unanimously demand for the immediate issuance of Antyodaya ration cards for the differently-abled citizens in India in the coming session of the Parliament as a step towards establishing food security. This would amount to a better recognizing of the rights of these people, especially in terms of their right to food security.[8]
- **Disable Friendly Buildings**: The courts in India have time and again directed the PWD, UDD and other departments concerned to file affidavits on facilities for disabled persons at public buildings across the different states in the country. The facilities should be designed in such a way that the differently abled persons do not get deprived with regards to accessibility to public places.[9] The infrastructure projects should be all-inclusive and incorporate utilities for the disabled, including ramps, toilets and separate parking space for the disabled. E.g. in the State of Karnataka, a scheme for 3 per cent reservation in allocation of houses and preferential treatment given to the same does exist. However in practicality this has been poorly implemented.[10]
- **Insurance Policies:** In response to a public interest litigation field by an impaired professor with regards to seeking parity with the general employees in terms of benefits, the Central government submitted that equal benefits for postal life

insurance will be provided to the differently-abled government employees with a maximum limit of Rs 5,00,000. Thus similar steps are also being taken to facilitate insurance policies to differently abled people.

- **Right to Education**: In addition to the Right to Education Bill which creates space for differently abled students, the CBSE has published a circular, for "individual evaluation programme" for special children based on their abilities and skill sets. Since special children may not be able to focus on the teacher during classroom interactions, and their pace of learning may be at variance with the rest of the class, schools have been told to allow a parent or aide to sit with the child in class and motivate him to "move along with the rest of the class". By making the class X boards optional, these mechanisms can be better implemented as the obsession of students and teachers with marks would reduce. However the parents of the disabled students are still skeptic as to whether the teachers equipped to deal with special kids? Do schools have the infrastructure and training to implement such a policy?[11]
- **Cyber Tools**: The Central government set up the Indian Accessibility Guidelines (IAG) in February 2009, a decision that mandates that no new government website would be created without following the rules such as: website to be equipped with alternate text for images, menus that can be operated with any input texts, such as through keyboards, joysticks and on-screen keyboards, provisions for learning through icons and accessing structured text under several simplified heads, captions for audio-video files allow hearing impaired users to navigate through the site and for the elderly or for those suffering from colour blindness, the site should have provisions for larger text size, contrast colours and wider spacing between words to reduce clutter. These state-of-art norms have been created in tune with international standards yet the government has not been very successful in implementing it thoroughly.[12] The government is also

contemplating to amend Copyrights Act in India to bring in publication of disabled friendly books.

- **Linkage between Disability and IT**: Similarly, understanding the issue of disability and its link with IT, NASSCOM recently instituted a Disability Advisory Group (DAG) wing. Text size, contrast, audio-video formats, and assistive devices are some of the considerations on which the group's agenda would focus on, keeping in mind factors of accessibility, employability and assistive technologies. Emphasis was laid on the use of Web Content Access Guidelines (WCAG) to make the worldwide web more accessible to all.[13]
- **Role of Media**: The role of media in sensitizing this issue has been laudable. Recently, the 'IBN7 Bajaj Allianz Super Idols' launched a first-of-its-kind initiative by a media organisation that pays tribute to the triumph of the human spirit over physical challenges and constraints in achieving greatness.[14] Some of the movies that have sought to enhance the sensitivity of society towards the needs, rights, sensibilities and potential of people with disabilities are—Sparsh, Black, Koshish (both old and new), Jagriti, Dosti, Main Aisa hi hun, Main Aisa Kyon Hun and Koi Mil Gaya. They have demonstrated the attempt of non-disabled people to understand people with disabilities.
- **Role of technology**: Recently, Shah Rukh Khan starrer, *My Name Is Khan* has become the first Bollywood film to be released in cinemas across the country with Hindi audio description (AD) for visually challenged people. AD provides narration that fits between passages of dialogue to describe action sequences, body language, costume and scenery, allowing the viewer to understand exactly what is happening on screen.[15]

Conclusion

Physical or mental disability is a silent crisis that not only affects the disabled persons and their families but also the social and economic development of entire society. Several kinds of discriminations are meted out to the disabled at different levels for no fault of their own. Poverty further adds to their woes. The poor people lack means for prevention and early detection of disability. Consequently, disabled are found disproportionately among the poorest strata of society. There are an estimated 600 million disabled in the world, of which around 350 million are in the developing countries. In India the accurate number of the disabled has not been assessed. The Sample Survey conducted in 1991 by the National Sample Survey Organisation (NSSO) estimated that about 1.9 per cent of the population of the country was disabled. The prevalence of physical disability was 20 per thousand persons in rural areas and 16 per thousand persons in urban areas. The fresh cases of disability every year have been estimated to be 7.5 lakh. By such estimates the disabled population must have grown tremendously. On an average, five per cent of the population is estimated to be suffering from some kind of disability.[16]

Since antiquity, society has detected disabilities arising out of obvious deficits in anatomical structures, sensory functions and intellectual developments amongst its members. These disabilities debarred the affected persons from participating in the mainstream of social life. With the decline of feudalism and the rise of democracy, the spirit of Zeitgeist favoured the concept of equal opportunity for care, employment, relief and empowerment for the disabled people. But the general view about what constitutes disability remained static for a very long time. Thanks to the recent spurt in the growth of scientific knowledge in this area and globalisation of the message of scientific activism, the concept of disability has become an important issue for re-examination and re-definition.[17]

Thanks to the growing legal and policy interventions that a community which was socially ostracized since time immemorial has been able to curve out a niche for itself through consistent movement and concern of their family members and social workers. Such responses have come a long way to provide a modicum of rights to be human to the community of disabled. The laws and policies though have been created with positive outlook but those at the helm of affairs seems to have lack of vision as they could not visualize the problem in its totality and make the laws and policies increasingly inclusive. Consequently, these laws and policies are requires to be amended in the light of changing nature of disability, growth in the field of science and technology and ever increasing population of disabled owing to environmental change; and intra-state and inter-state conflict which leads to man-made disability.

There is no denying the fact that something has been done and something has been happening, however, tremendous requires to be done. It makes it imperative that the union and state governments and policy makers in the country should brainstorm to overhaul the existing legal provisions to make it increasingly inclusive. Moreover, both laws and policies requires to be implemented in letter and spirit as true to Indian situations most sacrosanct and effective laws and policies fails at the stage of implementation. Therefore, alongside the amendment of the legal provisions major emphasis and monitoring is required to be done at the stage of implementation. As discussed above, media too has been playing a positive role and it must continue to do so with more vigor. Education institutions and Non-Governmental Organisations owe a greater responsibility in this field: First, towards raising the scale of awareness about the concerns of disabled; and second by coming forward with plans and actions to adopt them and make an effort to bring them into the mainstream of Indian society and polity.

Legal regimes are essential; however, there is also the need to change the mindset of common and able people through education and awareness program about the rights of the disabled. Such an effort would bear more fruit and would help more efficaciously towards addressing the problem in any society. Therefore, alongside the legal and policy intervention the government and others should try to educate the common masses about the concerns of the disabled or differently-abled as they have come to be addressed. Disabled or differently-abled are equal and free citizens of free India. Indian Constitution which is the fundamental law of the land does not make any distinction among the citizens of the country and duly protects the rights of the citizens.

REFERENCES

1. Prakriti SInghania, "Wind Beneath his Sails", *The Times News Network*, Jan 30, 2010.

2. http://www.worldbank.org.in/WBSITE/EXTERNAL/COUNTRIES/SOUTHASIAEXT/INDIAEXTN/0,,contentMDK:21557057~pagePK:1497618~piPK:217854~theSitePK: 295584,00.html (last visited 28.02.2010).
3. Bacquer and Sharma (1997); Coleridge (1993), Miles (1995) and Erb and Harriss-White (2002).
4. Prassana Kumar, "The Ability Debates", *India Together,* February 22, 2008.
5. "Impact of the Disability Convention on Indian domestic law" *Law Review–Action Aid* Sep. 2007 also available at http://www.indlaw.com/actionaid/?Guid=15df6a97-fc94-46e4-b567-e2e29c56a215 (last visited on 28.02.2010).
6. Aarti Dhar,"Move to make obtaining disability certificate easier", *The Hindu* (New Delhi), Feb 12, 2010.
7. Chitra Paul, "Simpler Disabilty Rules",*The Times of India* (New Delhi), Jan 14, 2010.
8. "Issue Antyodaya ration cards to differently abled", *The Hindu* (Kolkata), Feb 21, 2010.
9. "HC: are public buildings friendly to the disabled", *The Time of India* (New Delhi), Jan 14, 2010.
10. "Govt. takes 14 yrs for first review of Disability Act", *Deccan Herald* (Bangalore), Jan 12, 2010.
11. Anahita Mukherji, "Take special kids or face action: CBSE", *The Times of India,* Feb 4, 2010.
12. Swati Mathur, "Despite govt order, websites for disabled still a rarity", *The Times of India* (New Delhi), Jan 26, 2010.
13. Ramya Kannan, "Nasscom's disabled-friendly initiative gets ecstatic welcome", *The Hindu,* Jan 31, 2010.
14. "IBN7 Super Idols: People who've overcome adversity", *IBN-News,* Jan 11, 2010.
15. "MNIK first Hindi film with audio description", *NDTV News,* Jan 24, 2010.
16. India 2001 Figures.
17. Banerjee, G. (2001), "The Concept of Disability and Mental Illness", www.psyplexus.com/excel/cdmi.html visited on February 27, 2004.

9

Disabilities and Human Rights of Army Personnel

Anil Bhat

Mankind has never been kind enough to its own beings disabled since birth, or by sickness, or injury. Whether they are on the streets, or our own kith and kin, we as the human race have not collectively, or individually, been sensitive enough about nuances of disabilities and the kinds of problems that come with them. While in earlier days, rulers in their pursuit of power used torture as a modus to subdue rivals, even if they were of their own blood, in these modern times, with great advances in technologies, as the human race, we have not improved enough to ensure allotment of best available facilities and with wide reach for a daily increasing count of unfortunate people, who get maimed because of arson or calamity.

However, at least most countries have instituted systems to support disabled people. In India, where the government reserves a quota for scheduled castes and tribes, as well as some categories of disabled, there is much more that needs to be done for their rehabilitation. NGOs in this field, sponsored or financed by government, have contributed and more such may be welcome, but we need to keep striving to inform and inspire both the disabled and able-importantly, the well-placed amongst the latter.

Infringement of human rights is a serious problem the world over, but unfortunately, of the many NGOs in this field, not all can claim to be sincere and objective. An example is of many myths disproved, and many 'chickens come to roost' factors that emerged since 9/11. India was one of the countries, which despite suffering from Pakistan's India-Kashmir fixated and other-alignments-related nurturing and export of terrorism, and, ironically, its principled but very soft approach, kept getting unduly lambasted by Western countries. The post-9/11 period has almost jerked many in the world to look at India anew. Further, it is indeed ironic that the same countries which use to be so judgmental about India's record of human rights abuses, have beaten it hollow in the process of committing excesses while fighting global terrorism without any success.

While recording of history has been one of our weaknesses, lack of a sense of it seems to be even more so, although we remain great at creating it. The fact remains that for over 60 years since independence, important aspects of history, which have a direct bearing on present-day developments and will continue to bear on future ones, 20th century history of India is still not taught in its schools. But that does not absolve human rights related NGOs from presenting mostly one side of the picture—that of militants and terrorists—and branding the government and all security forces as suppressive.

It needs to be known that concern for the disabled started with World War I. Public concern in the West for the disabled started when disabled soldiers were demobbed from the armed forces and they had to beg on the streets for their living. This movement accelerated after WW I. Once the soldiers were attended to, then society turned their attention to other types of disability.

Let us take a brief look at post-Independence Indian history. There have been three conventional wars with Pakistan at the latter's instance-1947-48, 1965 and 1971. What has been happening in Jammu and Kashmir (J&K) since the late 1980s is low intensity war with export of terrorism by Pakistan. In 1962, there was a war with

China, with a lesser level repeat in 1967. Indian security forces, particularly Army, have been fighting insurgencies in North-Eastern states, which since early 1990s, degenerated into terrorism, thanks largely to Pakistan's ISI. Punjab was targeted by Pakistan with 'Khalistani' terrorism, which lasted for a decade at least and is now again being attempted to be revived again by ISI. Despite the peace process with Pakistan since November 2003, ISI continues to export terrorism in J&K foment dissent and bloodshed throughout India. Then there was the Indian Peace Keeping Forces' stint in Sri Lanka, a large number of peace keeping missions with the United Nations since its inception and many humanitarian disaster-relief actions undertaken every year since Independence.

In all these wars, conflicts and humanitarian operations many personnel died and of the injured, many got maimed permanently. Just the Indian Army's fatal casualties since 1947 till August 2005 have been 20852, whereas non-fatal have been over 21043. Of those surviving, almost 1000 are permanently disabled, with about 70 per cent of them being amputees, few of which lost more than one limb. Having interacted with many of Indian Army's disabled personnel, all I can say is that they are a tribute to the human spirit, from whom the physically fit could learn a lot. I will never forget Naik (an Indian Army non-commissioned rank) Narendra Singh of the 4th Battalion, of the Grenadiers Regiment, who lost both lower limbs as a result of grenades being hurled at him while fighting against Pakistani terrorists in J&K, during one of the peak years (1993). Anti-personnel mines during conventional wars and other indigenous explosive devices (IEDs) used by terrorists have accounted for a large number of loss of limb, sight or other kinds of disabilities.

Major General (retired) Ian Cardozo, SM, VSM (recipient of the Sena Medal for bravery and the Ati Vishishtha Seva Medal, for distinguished service of a high order by the President of India), who lost a lower limb owing to a minefield injury during the 1971 India-Pakistan War, heads the War Wounded Association of India and has also devoted a lot of time and effort towards philanthropic projects for disabled people.

Disabilities Rehabilitation and Human Rights of Armed Force Personnel in J&K

The concessions and facilities available to children of Defence personnel killed or disabled in action:

(a) Free educational facilities to children of Defence personnel killed or disabled in action;
(b) 25 seats in the MBBS, one seat in BDS and two seats in Engineering are available through KSB to dependants/wards of certain categories of Defence personnel as Government of India nominees;
(c) 25 per cent seats are reserved for the wards of serving and ex-Service personnel in Sainik Schools;
(d) reservation of seats in professional colleges/ITI/Polytechnics by various States/UTs for wards of serving and retired Defence personnel; and
(e) education grant of Rs 600 and Rs 300 p.m. per student to wards of war-bereaved, disabled, attributable and non-attributable peace time casualties respectively, housed in 35 War Memorial Hostels to pursue their studies.

Artificial Limb Centre, Pune. Since Independence, over 30,000 casualties of the Armed Forces have been treated here.

St Dunstan's After Care Organisation, Dehradun. The institution provides rehabilitation training financial support and psychological support to blinded serving personnel and ex-servicemen. This is funded by Kendriya Sainik Board and Oxford University Press, Delhi. A contribution of Rs 4 Lakh from the Army and Rs 1 lakh each by Navy and Air Force was provided to the institution in 2001 for setting up a corpus fund.

Queen Mary Technical Institute, Pune. The institute conducts ITI recognised vocational training for disabled servicemen and their dependents. The institute is funded out of grants from various Govt and Non-Govt agencies, AG's Branch and from Corpus Fund of the institute. Courses conducted by the institute commence on 1 August. Applications from serving personnel are processed through CW-5 section of Ceremonials and Welfare Directorate and the Directorate

General of Re settlement. Various disciplines in which the courses are conducted are as under:

- Fitter, electrician and radio/TV mechanic courses of two years duration.
- Diesel mechanic course of one year duration.
- Stenography (English) course of one year duration.
- Cutting and tailoring course of one year duration.

Paraplegic Homes. Paraplegic Rehabilitation Centres (PRC) at Kirkee and Mohali with a capacity of 80 and 30 beds respectively are being run for rehabilitation of paraplegic and tetraplegic ex-servicemen. These are being run as charitable trusts registered with the respective state government. In addition to these, a case is being processed with the Ministry of Defence for release of grant for establishing a Paraplegic Home at Lucknow. A vocational training centre has been established near Paraplegic Home Mohali for rehabilitation training of paraplegics. These institutions are funded by Kendriya Sainik Board, Ministry of Social Justice and Empowerment, AG's Branch and other state Government/private organisations. Postal address of PRC Kirkee and Mohali are as under:

Grants to disabled

	Officers	**JCOs/OR**
Ex-Gratia from Central Govt	Nil	
NDF (Applicable Only if Boarded out of Service): $		
75% to 100% disability	Rs 6 lakhs	Rs 6 lakhs.
50% to 75% disability	Rs 4.5 lakhs	Rs 4.5 lakhs
for less than 50% disability	Rs 3 lakhs	Rs 3 lakhs
Dwelling Units	Rs 5 lakhs	Rs 5 lakhs
Education (Max)(Rupees one lakh per child)	Rs 1 to 2 lakhs	Rs 1 to 2 lakhs
ACWF# (Based on % disability)	Rs 30,000	Rs 30,000

Note: $ Announced & Implemented w.e.f. Sept. 1999.
Announced & Implemented w.e.f. Oct. 1999.

Benefits to Disabled

Ex-Gratia from Central Govt	Nil
NDF	Nil
ACWF: # Boarded Out	Rs 1 Lakh
Retained in Service (Based on % disability)	Rs 30,000, Rs 20,000 or Rs 10,000.

Note: #Announced & Implemented w.e.f. Oct. 1999.

Army Welfare Housing Organization reserves 3 per cent of the dwelling units for allotment to war widows.

It is a pity that the above details of grants to the disabled grants to the disabled, according to some war-veterans, give quite a rosy picture. The facts are otherwise, e.g., the war disabled, earlier to Kargil, were not granted anything from the State or Central Governments.

Benefits for Disabled Soldiers Retained in Service. If disability is assessed at 20 per cent or more for life, the personnel are given an option for taking lump sum compensation in lieu of war injury pension equal to the capitalised value calculated at the following rates for 100 per cent disablement (these rates will proportionately reduce for lesser degree of disablement): Officers – Rs 2600 pm., Junior Commissioned Officers – Rs 1900 pm., and Other Ranks – Rs 1550 pm.

Major Offers for All Battle Casualties

Pepsi Co India Holding Ltd. The company has offered 500 Kiosks for allotment to NOK of soldiers killed in action and to war disabled soldiers. Salient aspects of the offer are as under : Kiosks are put up and maintained at the company's cost. Cooling equipment may be provided free of cost (Special cases). Company to service Kiosks on bi-weekly basis. Products of other companies can also be sold in these Kiosks.

Note: Applications for allotments of Kiosks are processed through

Rehabilitation and Welfare Section (R&W Sec.) of Ceremonial and Welfare Directorate (CWD) and forwarded to the Company.

STD/ISD PCOs. Department of Telecommunication allots PCOs on liberal terms to following categories of personnel :

- Widows or Dependents.
- Disabled Personnel or one of their dependents.
- Dependents of soldiers in captivity or missing in action.
- Educational Qualification in case of War Widows should be minimum 5th standard.

Note: Application for PCO booths may be forwarded by eligible personnel directly to Regional Managers of Telecommunication Department.

National Human Rights Commission has been able to secure relief by way of ex-gratia compensation to the next of kin of a victim of the militant attack at Kaluchak in Jammu & Kashmir on 14 May 2002. A complaint was filed on 20 October 2003 by Shri J.N. Yadav who stated that he has served in the Army since last 30 years. He said that on 14 May 2002, three unidentified armed terrorist attacked an army camp at Kaluchak, J&K which caused heavy casualties. During the said attack, the terrorists killed/injured three of his family members which included his wife Premvati Devi who died and his sons Krantivir Singh and Virat Singh who were left with disabilities. He further stated that the incident has left him totally shaken, as his small family had been broken. He prayed for grant of financial assistance.

Upon receiving the petition, the Commission directed that a copy of the complaint be sent to the Secretary, Ministry of Defence, Government of India, New Delhi and Chief Secretary, Jammu & Kashmir to look into the allegations contained in the complaint and to submit their comments within four weeks.

A communication dated 4 February 2004 was received from the Ministry of Defence, Government of India with a report on the grant of ex-gratia compensation to the next of kin of the deceased members of family of Defense Service Personnel. The report inter-alia stated that the instances and the amount that could be given as ex-gratia to next of kin of the deceased Defence Service Personnel who die in harness in the performance of bona fide duties in cases are: where death occurred due to accidents in the course of performance of duties the compensation is Rs.5.00 lakh, if death occurred/due in the course of performance of duties attributable to acts of violence by terrorists, anti-social elements the compensation is Rs.5.00 lakh, in death occurring during border skirmishes and action against militants, terrorists, extremists etc, the amount is Rs.7.5 lakh, and in death occurring during enemy action in international war or such war like engagements which are specifically notified by Ministry of Defence, it is Rs. 10.00 lakh.

It stated that there is no provision that covers ex-gratia compensation where the members of the family of defence service personnel are killed in such a situation as the militant attack in Kaluchak. But the State Government of J&K has been providing ex-gratia relief/compensation to the victims of militancy/cross firing for death, injury etc. to the next of kin of the deceased. As per the State Government orders Rs.1.00 lakh is paid to the next of kin in case of death, Rs.75,000, Rs.5,000 and Rs.1,000 for permanent disability, grievous injury and minor injury respectively, caused in terrorist incidents. The said expenditure of the State Government in this regard is being reimbursed by the Central Government. It stated that compensation of Rs.1.00 lakh has already been sanctioned in 18 cases of death by the State Government by their order dated 17 October 2002. The name of late Smt. Premvati Devi, it stated, has been covered in the said list. The details regarding financial relief to Master Krantivir Singh and Master Virat Singh who were injured/disabled in the said incident are being ascertained from Department of J&K Affairs, Ministry of Home Affairs. The Home Department, Government of J&K later communicated to the Commission that ex-gratia relief amounting to Rs.1.00 lakh has been sanctioned by the Deputy Commissioner, Jammu on 17 October 2002. It said that Rs. 1.00 lakh has been paid through the G.O.C. Tiger Division, Jammu to the next of kin of Premvati Yadav, W/o Sub. Jagdish Narayan. Further, the ex-gratia amount of Rs.75,000 and Rs.5,000 has also been sanctioned by the Deputy Commissioner, Jammu on

8 July 2003 and paid in favour of Krantivir Siangh and Virat Singh, sons of J.N. Yadav who were disabled and injured due to militants firing at Kaluchak on 14 May 2002. The sanctioned amount has been paid to them through the said G.O.C.

Mukesh Anand (warwounded@yahoo.co.uk), Executive Director-WAR WOUNDED FOUNDATION and President- MISSION VIJAY-2, has since 2000, resettled or rehabilitated a large number of war-wounded and war-widows. Details of some of them are:

L.Hav. Suleman—18 JK Rif (09427050587) of Vill–Aderan Po–Navavas Distt–Banaskantha (Gujarat), received bullet injury in knee during an operation at Kupwara in July-2003. GUJARAT AMBUJA CEMENT- w.e.f. 8.04.2006. Invested Rs. 50000 and sold 50 bags within two days.

Sep. N.K. Desmane—BEG Kirki (09822214241) Satara Distt (MS) sustained mine blast injury in 1965 war. Started INDIAN OIL LUBS w.e.f. 8.4.2006. Invested 13000 rupees.

Hav Nirmal Singh-4 Sikh (09417088526) VPO Dasuya, Hoshiarpur (PB). Bullet injury in right hand. License for selling Fertilizer issued to him 2.4.2006. Started Chambal Fertilizer dealership w.e.f. 10.4.2006. Received two truck supply and Invested Rs. 100000.

(For further details kindly contact National Human Rights Commission, Faridkot House, Copernicus Marg, New Delhi, PIN 110001 Tel. No. 23382742, Fax No. 23384863, E-Mail: covdnhrc @nic.in, ionhrc@nic.in)

Here are some details about disabled soldiers:

36 year-old Rajendran is a army veteran with an artificial leg and blinded in one eye. Four years ago, fighting terrorists in the mountainous area of Jammu & Kashmir, a Pakistani artillery shell nearly killed him. Slowly, he is learning to start life afresh at a rehabilitation school for battle-maimed army veterans in the idyllic Deccan plateau of western India.

Wheelchair-bound Kumudchandra Saikia, 38, is also learning how to operate a computer at the Queen Mary's Technical Institute For Disabled Soldiers (QMTI) in Khadki on the outskirts of Pune.

While the above two entries are from internet, The Week magazine (February 27, 2011) published a feature about disabled personnel, who have not been given the kind or level of compensation commensurate with the nature of their disabilities:

In June 1988, 54 years old Naib Subedar Balu Ram Nehra lost his left eye to fragments from a grenade, when he was with the Indian Peace Keeping Force (IPKF) in Sri Lanka. He gets Rs. 9000 as pension from the government which does not meet his family needs and survives by farming his 11 bighas.

Havildar Sajjan Singh Yadav also became disabled while fighting the LTTE in Sri Lanka. All his muscles below his waist are dead. He gets a pension of Rs. 10,000 from the government which is not enough for him to survive as more than half is waved away for his medicines.

Naik Ashok Kumar is paralysed in one leg after a shell broke and was followed by a bullet hit which broke his helmet and knocked him down. He earns his living by practicing yoga as the Rs. 10,200 pension from the government is insufficient for him.

Naik Dharamveer Yadav lost his left hand and right eye during action against Pakistan Army. He was declared completely disabled by the Army medical board and got a compensation of only Rs. 2.20 lacs. "At that time I got Rs. 2.20 lakh only. Even today I have not got my full pension. Is this the cost of a hand and an eye just Rs. 2 lakh? Is this the cost of serving my motherland?" he is quoted to have said.

Havildar Rang Lal was shot in his left leg by Pakistan army on the Line of Control in Mendhar, Jammu & Kashmir. He is unable to walk and does not receive any pension.

Naik Surendra Kumar lost his left leg while fighting against Pakistani troops in operation Vijay (Kargil War in 1999). He is most dissatisfied with the disability pension and the treatment from the government as well as the Army.

Tabled below are figures of Indian Army personnel killed and injured in operations mostly against Pakistan army or terrorists supported by it from 1990 till early 2011.

Year	Death	Injured
1990	155	332
1991	173	520
1992	189	715
1993	198	897
1994	200	773
1995	237	789
1996	189	542
1997	216	390
1998	268	479
1999	407	741
2000	482	864
2001	613	1587
2002	539	1085
2003	384	814
2004	330	651
2005	244	433
2006	182	848
2007	122	336
2008	135	180
2009	79	130
2010	69	965
2011	02	02

The conflict are on increase since last many decades and are expected to continue in foreseeable future. Indian State is also getting mighty, therefore, they have to contain the conflicts in this process violence is escalating and leaving a large pool of disabled people in general and in security forces in particular. The security forces and government of India have involved the mechanism to cope with the situation. However, more concrete measures must be taken in order to protect the comprehensive rights of the disables.

10

Disability and Judiciary

P. Saibabu and C. Ravi Sankar

The 1970s marked a new approach to disability. The concept of human right for disabled persons began to become more accepted internationally. The declaration of the rights of the disabled persons adopted by the General Assembly on 9th December 1975 encouraged national and international protection of the rights of the disabled. Recognition was given to the fact that disabled persons were entitled to the same political and civil rights as others, including measures to enable them to become self sufficient. The declaration reiterated the rights of disabled persons to education, medical services, and placement service. It further recognized their right to economic and social security, employment, to live with their families, to participate in social and creative events, to be protected against all exploitation, abuse or degrading behavior, and to avail them of legal aid. Realizing the need to promote the full participation of the disabled in the social life and development of their societies, on 16th December 1976, the General Assembly declared the year 1981 International Year of Disabled Persons (IYDP), stipulating that it be devoted to integrating disabled persons fully in to society.

There are 500 million persons with disabilities worldwide (or) 10 percent of the global population. Approximately two thirds live in developing countries. In certain developing countries nearly 20 percent of the general population is in some way disabled; if the impact on their families is taken into account, 50 percent of the population is affected.

India has an estimated population of the disabled 9 cores. The census 2001 estimations is not perfect due to various reasons for which there is no proper scientific base However the 9 core disabled population demands for their rights and full participation in all aspects of their life. Mostly the human rights are being violated in terms of education, training and employment, public transport, public buildings, housing and other social and cultural areas. In order to overcome the barriers necessary study must be conducted and low attempt has been made in this regard. The number of disabled persons continues to increase in tandem with growth of the world population. Factors causing the increase in their number include war and other forms of violence, inadequate medical care, and natural and other disasters.

Not surprisingly, many of the disabled are poor. The overwhelming majority- perhaps 80 percent live in isolated rural areas. Almost that many live in areas where the services needed to help them are unavailable. Too often their lives are handicapped by physical and social barriers in society, which hamper their full participation. Because of this, and in all parts of the world, they often face a life that is segregated and debased and without help many will live in isolation and insecurity. "Disability is not a tragedy, it's an inconvenience".

The World Health Organization, in its International Classification of Impairments, Disabilities and Handicaps, makes a distinction between impairment, disability and handicap. These three concepts are defined by it as follows:

(a) Impairment is "any loss or abnormality of psychological, physiological, or anatomical structure or structure of function". Impairments are disturbances at the level of the organ which includes defects in or loss of a limb, organ or other body structure as well as defects in or loss of a mental function. Examples of impairments include blindness, deafness, loss of sight in an eye, paralysis of a limb, amputation of a limb; mental retardation, partial sight, loss of speech, autism.

(b) Disability is a "restriction or lack (resulting from an impairment) of ability to perform an activity in the manner or within the range considered normal for a human being". It describes a functional limitation or activity restriction caused by impairment. Disabilities are descriptions of disturbances in function at the level of the person. Examples of disabilities include difficulty seeing, speaking or hearing; difficulty moving or climbing stairs; difficulty grasping, reaching, bathing, eating, toileting.

(c) A handicap is a "disadvantage for a given individual, resulting from an impairment or disability that limits or prevents the fulfillment of a role that is normal (depending on age, sex and social and cultural factors) for that individual". The term is also a classification of "circumstances in which disabled people are likely to find themselves". Handicap describes the social and economic roles of impaired or disabled persons that place them at a disadvantage compared to other persons. These disadvantages are brought about through the interaction of the person with specific environments and cultures. Examples of handicaps include being bedridden or confined to home; being unable to use public transport; being socially isolated.

There are serious human rights violations in India in general, more so in the case of disabled persons. The disabled person's rights are not fully recognized up to 1995. As a result of the pressure from the United Nations, Declaration of as IYDP the year 1981, the UN Decade from 1983-93 and the internal agitations by various disabled elite disabled groups in India, the Government of India enacted a law in partial fulfillment of the rights of the disabled in India in the year 1995 **[The Persons with Disabilities (equal opportunities, protection of rights and full participation) Act, 1995]**.

Even after the Parliamentary enhancement of 1995 act, the Policy makers and the implementing agencies did not implement the Law in its true spirit. The rights that are promised by the law a few individuals, associations, NGOs approached the Honorable courts in protecting their rights. Due to lack of time and other reasons, we present a few cases of such kind where the rights are protected and guaranteed their opportunities by various judgments.

Few Judgements

In the case *Indira Sahani* Vs *Union of India* properly has known as Mandal case. The famous Supreme Court Judgment for providing reservations to the Backward Classes covered under Article 16(4) of the Constitution of India. In this case defining the word Backwardness the Apex court categorically stated that the Backwardness means economic backwardness, social, educational and physically backwardness. The physically backwardness itself an implied meaning of that the disabled persons are also covered by the Constitution who are disserved to get their rights such as employment, education and social security and so on, but the problem in this case is the court has fixed that under no circumstances the percentage of reservations should not exceed 50 per cent, 22 per cent for SCs and STs and 27 per cent for BCs, total percentage is 49½ is prescribed by the court. The court did not clarify how to provide 3 per cent reservation to the disabled. This question is still left unanswered. The fate of the disabled is left at the mercy of the Government for providing reservations.

There is another remarkable case *Social Jurist, a lawyers' Group* Vs *Government of Delhi and Anr.*, in its nature if we ask why the answer is very simple. The Constitution of India has provided some guidelines to provide education to all children irrespective of caste, color, and creed. Providing education is implied that constructions of School buildings and provide peaceful atmosphere to pursue this education under Article 41 of the Constitution. The government is to provide education to vulnerable sections, such as disabled. This idea is further elaborated in article 45 of the Constitution which provides compulsory education to all the children below the age of

14. This idea has categorically given its conclusion that all children including physically challenged.

In a case on providing food security to the people of India under right to life under the article 21 of Constitution of India, the Government of India has started public distribution scheme under which subsidiaries like rice and wheat are being supplied to all the people, who are under below poverty line. The notable point in this case is 95 per cent of the physically challenged are from among their poor. The term below poverty line directly indicates that scheme of the food security should be extended to the physically challenged unconditionally. But this is being not done in a proper manner on which Government should take some steps for providing food security to the physically challenged.

Education is a basic fundamental right. The right has been recognized disabilities act 1995. The importance of section 39 came into light with the case filed by *All Kerala Parents Association of impaired* Vs *State of Kerala*. In this case the parents of hearing impaired challenged the Government action for not providing medical education to their children under section 39 of Disabilities action in Kerala High Court. The Kerala High Court has accepted the Government action under the contention that section 39 of afore said act is only related to the employment but not to the education. The court is not in position to reject the Governments plea under the section which is not about the education. But Apex Court of India has questioned the Judgment. The court is of the opinion that section 39 is broad in its nature but providing education only the Government can provide the employment, so we can not bifurcated the two rights from one to another. Under the section the Government is under obligation that it should not deny the right of education of the physically challenged under the contention of the meaning of a section by interrupting of its own meaning.

Regarding the Human rights of disability, the need for providing rights particularly the right to education, which is self support in this process in a case *Dr. Raman Khanna and others* Vs *University of Delhi*, the Delhi High Court has rejected the guidelines issued by Medical Counsel of India and the Delhi University inviting applications form physically challenged for the admissions in Medical colleges. These guidelines are highly objective in their own nature, because of giving criteria to the percentage of disability from 40 per cent to 70 per cent that means the higher degree of disabled are not suitable for the admissions. The Delhi High Court has ordered the Delhi University and Medical Counsel of India to give priority to the higher degree of disability in the medical colleges as per the Act of disability 1995.

The Delhi High Court did not mention the distribution of reservation quota i.e. 3 per cent in the absence of one category or the other which is not suitable to take up the course. For an instance the Visually Handicapped are not suitable to get the admissions in the medical colleges. In such a case the 1 per cent grant quota of visually challenged should be allotted to other categories which are in race.

In continuation of providing right to education has brought out an innovative case i.e. *Dhawal S. Choti* Vs. *Union of India & others*, regarding providing extra time in examinations to the physically challenged, which cannot compete in writing with their general counter parts. A persons suffering from cerebral palsy requested the authorities to grant three hours extra time for him to write the Intermediate examination of Charted Accounting. But the authorities have granted him only half-an-hour. But the court considering the importance of situation ordered the authorities to grant him extra time 3 hours which he is requested for the court here has done yeoman service by upholding the human rights pertaining to the disabled.

The right to education is continues process on which the arguments are being raised from time to time in different courts. In one case *The Government of Tamilanadu* Vs *Master J. Rajkumar (Minor)*, in this case the Tamilnadu court for the first time openly declares that all the provisions including section 39 of disabilities act are not directory but mandatory. The term mandatory denotes that all the Government bodies or the agencies should be abide by the disabilities acts without any failure.

In other case relating to the education to be provided fort the physically challenged particularly for visually challenged the court has directed the National Counsel for Training and Education to provide free education to visually challenged of their financial conditions and domicile conditions as requested by National Federation of the blind.

Regarding the right to education not only the India courts but also the Western courts have reacted sharply. The Supreme Court of United States of America has recognized the scheme of integrated education with a view to interning the handicapped with the non-handicapped. In other case providing education to all handicapped is an absolute duty of the Government. It has been recognized by the United States Supreme Court in Rowley's case.

The employment which is guaranteed by the Constitution of India and Disabilities Act, 1995, in a leading case between *Dayaram Tripathi* Vs *State of Uttar Pradesh and others*, a serious argument has been raised by the Uttar Pradesh Government, regarding the reservation of Jobs for handicapped. All the handicapped are not fit to discharge their duties in particular fields, in such posts it is not possible for the Government to provide reservations. Through series of letters and office memos the Uttar Pradesh Government has suspended the reservations for handicapped as suggested by the Uttar Pradesh Public Service Commission. The Government has canceled the reservations in Uttar Pradesh civil services which are not suitable for handicapped. Dayaram filed a writ petition in Allahabad High Court challenging the cancellation of reservations; meanwhile the year 1981 has been observed as International Year of Disabled Persons. The Government has accepted its moral duty on revaluated its earlier order providing 2 per cent reservation including the Uttar Pradesh Public Service Commission. Hence the court has also allowed the appeal and ordered the Government to continue the reservation policy without hindrance in future.

Article 32 of the Constitution of India is a wonderful boon to the citizens of India in general but visually handicapped in particularly. In a case *National Federation of Blind* Vs *Union Public Service Commission and others* highlights this issue. The National Federation of Blind has filed a writ petition in the Supreme Court seeking permission to appear for the Civil Services by the visually handicapped candidates. The National Federation of Blinds of their opinion though the visually handicapped people are well educated, though they are capable of discharging their duties with the help of a stenographer like others. But they are not given reservations in I.A.S. and allied services. The Apex court has allowed the writ petition and ordered the Government to make arrangements in this regard. Further the court has ordered to look into the matter of identification of Jobs for various categories of handicapped. According the Government has formulated a committee to look into the matter. The committee has identified 416 categories including allied services. But the visually challenged is frequently raising their voice against the discrimination shown to them by the Government. No, single person has been recruited so far as an I.A.S. officer. They are questioning the authorities of the Government allowing the visually challenged persons for civil services examinations without providing them 3 per cent reservations in I.A.S. and allied services. This question has been still under the carpet of discussion.

In a case in which a person suffering with color blindness was denied to be appointed as an officer in agricultural department of Maharashtra Government, because of his problem with vision. The appellant filed an affidavit before the court requesting to appoint him as an officer in agricultural department in 35 posts out of which only the 5 posts are required the perfect vision. He has countered the perfect remaining 30 posts need not require the perfect vision. Even the low vision persons can discharge the duties without any problem. The court allowed his appeal and ordered the Government to appoint him in any of the 30 posts which do not require the perfect vision s requested by the appellant. The court further mentioned in its order the entire appointment process should be completed with in 2 months from the date of receipt of orders by the concerned departments, This case clearly indicates that the modern Governments which are in way of escaping they obligations providing jobs to the handicapped on a small and petty cause or the problems being suffered by the handicapped. Even the principles of the natural justice are not being applied in case of handicapped whenever they approach the Head of the Departments to seek their redressal in future. The judiciary must be very strict in such cases and strict action may be initiated on these officials who deny the rights of handicapped.

Conclusion

In spite of the Constitutional provisions, the Equal Opportunities and Protection Act, 1995, and various judgments that are given by the Honorable courts, still there is a serious gap between the rural and urban, highly and low level educated, rich and poor, male and female, which itself reflect in the promise and performance of the state. To reduce that serious gap, the rights of the disabled are to be recognized as a part of the academic curriculum. There is every need to disseminate the information about the rights and opportunities by organizing Seminars, Workshops and Awareness programs by using all types of media at all levels at regular interval, so as to bring out a change in the social stigma.

REFERENCES

1. Constitution of India, New Delhi, 1950.
2. *Indira Sahani* Vs. *Union of India.*
3. *Dr. Raman Khanna and others* Vs. *University of Delhi.*

11

Parliament vis-à-vis Social Justice to Disabled Persons

S. Prabhakar

Introduction – Significance of Parliament

Parliament has a lot of say in engineering social justice. Of late, its role has come to the fore considerably. Parliament wields enormous power in ensuring accountability of the Ministry of Social Justice and Empowerment, through which various schemes for the disabled are executed. There is no denying of the fact that monitoring of various schemes by different actors in the scene is required. With the help of various weapons that are at its disposal, Parliament maintains a steady check on the Ministry and implementation of various programmes and plans aimed at empowering the Disabled to lead a honest and honourable live.

Parliament had enacted laws in connection with marriage, divorce, reservation, untouchability, labour, children, women, factories, atrocities, agriculture et al which had undoubtedly hastened the social justice to percolate deep into the weakest and vulnerable strata of society. It would not be an exaggeration to say that Parliament, along with State Assemblies contribute in bringing about social justice in multifarious fields.

It is stated that Legislature is an agency which determines the nature and aims of social justice. To deliver social justice to the people, first and foremost requisite is, people should be identified. Second comes the interests, needs and the problems of those people who are in need of social justice.

It is widely believed and accepted that law is an instrument of social justice. It is also believed that social justice must flow from the legal system as otherwise 'rule or law' will break down. Social justice includes welfare, and empowerment of disadvantaged and marginalized sections of the society, namely, Scheduled Castes, Aged persons, Persons with Disabilities, Backward Classes, Victims of Drug Abuse, etc.

Safeguards Provided in the Constitution

Article 14 of the Constitution guarantees that no person will be denied equality before the law. Articles 15, 16, 17 of the Fundamental Rights and Articles 38, 39, 39A, 41, 43, 43A and 46 of the Directive Principles, related to the various social, economic and political justice, getting inspiration from the protective umbrella of Article 31(C) and thus, contributing to the process of transformation in the society. It is not an exaggeration to state that 'social justice' and 'rule of law' are interdependent. Both have to go together in order to achieve justice, equality and freedom.

Under Article 253 to the Constitution of India read with item No.13 of the Union List, the Government of India enacted "The Persons with Disabilities (Equal Opportunities, Protection of Rights and Full Participation) Act, 1995."[1] This endeavour was to make sure that equal opportunities are given to the persons with disabilities and participation in the nation-building is full and complete.

Various constitutional provisions are there in the Constitution of India especially those which are relevant to social justice and empowerment, as highlighted above. For example, for security equality and justice, Constitution provides Parliament to enact laws, which citizens are expected to obey in order to achieve the aim for which the legal provisions are brought in. In this, the role of both the implementing agencies and common citizens is important. But in India, we have numerous religions, castes, customs, and above all different political parties. Under these circumstances, enacting laws is an arduous task. Parliament has the paramount duty and right to enact laws keeping in view the prevailing and developing economic and social circumstances. First and foremost, it has to keep in mind the requirement of the people. According to D.R. Jatava:

> "The religion-based legal system, which dominated the Indian society traditionally through the ages, has given way to the new legal system based on the Constitution. The divine origin of the social theory does not have any meaning in the present set-up. From the legal viewpoint, the significance of Varnashram Dharma carries no weight, no relevance, to the modern mind. However, there are certain religions, which have their `personal laws' such as the Muslim and Hindu laws. Some of these laws do not accord with the spirit of the Constitution and indirectly oppose the equality before law. Thus, the Indian legislatures have been entrusted with decisive roles in bringing about uniformity in our legal system."[2]

Various Acts have been passed in Parliament which aimed at extending reservation opportunities to certain classes to promote equality in the society or imparting social justice in different strata of society.

Before going into the nitty-gritty of the functionings of the Ministry, I would like to briefly state about the persons with disabilities. As per the 2001 Census, there are 2.19 crore.[3] They are 2.13 percent of the total population of the country. 'Persons with disabilities' include those who have visual, hearing, speech, locomotor and mental disabilities. According to the 58th Round of the National Sample Survey (NSS) of 2002, there were 208 lakh persons with disabilities in 2002 (Report No.485 at S.No.88). It is also stated that 75 per cent of such persons live in rural areas; 49 per cent of them is literate and only 34 per cent are employed. This is the sorry start of affairs. Hence, catering to their needs is indeed a tall order for the Government.

Ministry of Social Justice and Empowerment

Ministry of Social Justice and Empowerment is engaged in

coordination with different Ministries of the Central Government, State Governments/Union Territories, Central and State Public Sector Undertakings, local authorities and various other authorities for the implementation of various provisions of the Act. In spite of large-scale development in all most every sphere, particularly since 1991, we can find over 70 per cent of the population still living in the rural areas. In such a scenario, the task of the Government to dispense social justice has become arduous when such large chunk of population is deprived of basic necessities of life.

There is a separate Division called "Empowerment of Persons with Disabilities" in the Ministry of Social Justice and Empowerment. There are various schemes and programmes aimed at empowerment of persons with disabilities, namely, assistance to Disabled Persons for purchase/fittings of aids and appliances, Deendayal Disabled Rehabilitation Scheme to promote Voluntary Action for Persons with Disabilities, Scheme of National Awards for Empowerment of Persons with Disabilities, Scheme of National Scholarships for Persons with Disabilities, Trust Fund for Empowerment of Persons with Disabilities.

Apart from the above, there are a number of Schemes arising out of the Implementation of the Persons with Disabilities (Equal Opportunities, Protection of Rights and Full Participation) Act, 1995 – (a) Incentives to Employers in the Private Sector for Providing Regular Employment to Persons with Disabilities; (b) Models to promote awareness about accessibility features in public buildings; (c) Composite Regional Centres for Persons with Disabilities; (d) District Disability Rehabilitation Centres; (e) Awareness Generation Programme; and (f) Technology Development Projects in Mission Mode.

Ministry of Social Justice and Empowerment is the nodal Ministry to take care of social justice in all its aspects. National Commission for Scheduled Castes, National Commission for Backward Classes, National Commission for Safai Karmacharis, Rehabilitation Council of India, Babu Jagjivan Ram National Foundation, Dr. Ambedkar Foundation, National Backward Classes Finance and Development Corporation are some of the Commissions, Councils and Foundations under the Ministry.

Ministry extends assistance to Non-Governmental Organizations (NGOs) working for the welfare of disadvantaged sections of the society like Drug Addicts, Street Children, Disabled.[4]

Parliament's Use of Power for Securing Equality and Justice to the Persons with Disabilities

Parliament has a Departmentally-Related Standing Committee on Social Justice and Empowerment. It consists of 20 Members from Lok Sabha and 10 Members from Rajya Sabha. In the 14th Lok Sabha, Sumitra Maharan is the Chairperson of the Committee. From time to time, the Committee has been making recommendations to the Government.

Understanding the growing importance and growing awareness of the term 'social justice, the name of the Ministry of Welfare was changed to the Ministry of Social Justice and Empowerment in May, 1998. A whole lot of subjects are dealt by the Ministry, namely, social security, social insurance, providing relief to the disabled and unemployable; education, training and rehabilitation and welfare of the physically and mentally handicapped; promotion of efforts including voluntary efforts to ensure the well being of the older persons; educational and social welfare aspects of drug addition, etc.

In the 14th Lok Sabha, 930 questions were asked to seek information on various aspects of social justice and empowerment. Questions were as varied as Empowerment of the physically challenged persons, old age homes, transgender population, rehabilitation of physically challenged children, District Disability Rehabilitation Centres, employing the Disabled persons, monthly pension or ex-gratia to widows and handicapped, welfare schemes for disabled, welfare centres for Disabled Persons, Separate Budget for Disabled Persons, Public Transport Vehicle for Disabled, Central grants to NGOs, amendments to the Disability Laws, Disabled Children, employment of the Disabled in the Private Sector, National Policy for the Disabled People, Disabled People living in Hilly Tribal and Remote Areas.

Legal Framework

Four legislations have specially been directed towards the protection, welfare, rehabilitation and development of people with disabilities. They are – The Mental Health Act, 1987, Persons with Disabilities (Equal Opportunities, Protection of Rights and Full Participation) Act, 1995, The National Trust for Welfare of Persons with Autism, Cerebral Palsy, Mental Retardation and Multiple Disability Act, 1999 and the Rehabilitation Council of India Act, 1992.

A comprehensive National Policy for Persons with Disabilities has been announced in February, 2006, which recognized that disabled people are valuable human resources for the country. Policy aimed at primarily on prevention of disability, early detection and appropriate interventions, physical and economic rehabilitation measures, inclusive education, employment in the public and private sector and self-employment, creation of a barrier-free environment and development of rehabilitation professionals.

India has also ratified The United Nations Convention on the Rights of People with Disabilities (UNCRPD) in October, 2007, which enjoins upon India to ensure that all the rights enshrined in the Constitution, the current legislations, as well as UNCRPD, are speedily and effectively operationalized. In the 11th Plan, as India being a signatory of UNCRPD, it is obligatory on the part of India to incorporate the essence of Convention in our planning, implementation, monitoring and review processes.

Promoting Social Justice through Parliament

Now, let me turn to various ways in which parliament has taken upon itself to bring in social justice. The latest phenomenon which has entered the annals of parliament, in the 14th Lok Sabha, is setting up of different Parliamentary Forums. Namely –

1. Parliamentary Forum on Water Conservation and Management;
2. Parliamentary Forum on Youth—
    (a) Sub-Forum on Sports and Youth Development,

(b) Sub-Forum on Health,
(c) Sub-Forum on Education,
(d) Sub-Forum on Employment;

3. Parliamentary Forum on Children;
4. Parliamentary Forum on Population and Public Health.

The decision to set up Parliamentary Forums on different subjects was at the initiation of the Speaker, Lok Sabha, Somnath Chatterjee so that Members of Parliament can discuss the critical issues in a structured manner and also to raise the issue more effectively on the floor of the House.[5] These Forums would help the Members of Parliament to equip themselves and understand the issues in a better fashion. The broad aim and objective of these Fora are to equip the Members of Parliament with information and knowledge regarding issues and developments in different areas and also to make them aware of the seriousness of the situation and to enable them to adopt a result-oriented approach towards these issues.[6]

On the above lines, I would like to suggest here that a Parliamentary Forum on Social Justice should be set up to look into various aspects of social justice, including Persons with Disabilities, and to make sure the social justice is meted out to those who are in need of it the most.

Let me briefly touch upon the functions of these Forums. These Forums would focus their deliberations on strategies relating to respective problems; discuss and prepare strategies; build great awareness in all sections of the society, particularly at the grass-roots level; identify problems and make suggestions/recommendations for consideration and appropriate action by government/organizations concerned; identify the ways of involving Members of Parliament in these issues; organize seminars/workshops/orientation programmes, etc. to create awareness; to interact on a regular basis with concerned representatives and leaders in order to better appreciate their concerns and problems; to consider ways for improving Parliament's out-reach to different sections of society in order to reinforce their faith and commitment in democratic institutions and encourage their active participation therein; to provide a platform to Parliamentarians to exchange ideas, views, experiences, expertise, in a structured manner and to have an interface with civil society in highlighting concerned issues, including inter-alia, the voluntary sector, media and corporate sector and thereby to foster effective strategic partnerships in the concerned areas; hold comprehensive dialogue and discussion in respective matters with experts at the national and international levels and to have interactions with the multilateral organizations like WHO, UN agencies like UNICEF, etc., academicians, expert reports, studies, news and trend-analysis, etc. world-wide and concerned government agencies, which are germane to developments in the concerned sector.[7]

By the formation of above Forums, Parliament has turned a new leaf with the sole intention of addressing the major problems afflicting the nation in an organized manner with the help of experts opinion, with the invaluable inputs from the think-thank on the concerned field and acting as an appendage to Parliament, related Standing Committee and the Ministry helping. This would certainly add to the parliament's contribution to the democracy and nation building as it would take up the issues concerning a particular topic and fully and completely discuss and find a viable solution through its incisive and thought-provoking deliberations. Members of these Forums would have the benefit of expert advice and the assistance of think-tank in knowing fully the intricacies and complexities of the issue involved in these Forums, which would in turn help the Members to know the issue in its true sense to arrive at a solution and to form a considered opinion. This is a welcome step. This would only lessen the burden of the Ministries and Committees to a certain extent in dealing with the respective matters and would certainly help the Ministries and Committees to resolving the issues raised or taken up in these Forums.

In one's mind, an apprehension may arise about the clash of interests between the ministries/departments/committees on the one hand, and these Forums on the other hand. It has been made clear that the functioning of these Forums would not impinge on the ministries/departments/committees. The important and pressing issues concerning these Forums come up before Parliament often. Through these Forums, a sincere effort has been made to have a focused presentation of issues in Parliament, which would go a long way in knowing and understanding of the problems. This is the prime reason behind formation of these Forums on important topics.

BPST also holds Lectures and Seminars for Members of Parliament and of State Legislatures. It also organizes Orientation Programmes and Seminars for Media Personnel accredited to the Press Galleries of Parliament, apart from Training and Refresher Courses, Appreciation Courses for officers of Secretariats of Parliament and of State Legislatures in India and others. It also organizes Training, Attachment and Study Visits/tours of the Presiding Officers, Members and officers of foreign Parliaments and government officers, academics, scholars, students and others.[8]

Parliament wields enormous power in the governance of the country. The actions of government can be questioned and scrutinized by Parliament in its functioning. Parliament has been equipped with many constitutional provisions to rake up issues concerning the policies, schemes, programmes and plans of the government. These provisions should be made to more use to ensure that funds meant for the benefit of Disabled Persons and persons belong to vulnerable strata of society reach them and they reap the fruits of such programmes. The current trend of non-utilization of funds, return of funds allocated to the programmes meant for the upliftment of Disabled Persons should go.

So far, two Round Table Discussions have taken place under the aegis of Lok Sabha. Both Discussions were on 'Strengthening Parliamentary Democracy'. Here I would like to suggest that a Round Table Discussion should be attempted on the topic 'Rendering Social Justice'. Many eminent personalities should be invited to participate in the Discussion to strengthen the delivery mechanism of social justice across the country. Parliament has the statutory role to take the lead in dispensing social justice and to ensure that the laws which are in the statute book are implemented in letter and spirit. And those who take the laws in their own hands or those who do not strictly abide by the law, should be taken to task and should be penalized heavily. Parliament has a pivotal role to play here. Implementing agencies should understand the role of Parliament in its right perspective. Non-MPs too should be asked to participate in the discussions of the Parliamentary Forum on Social Justice. Forum should meet at regular intervals to take stock of the prevailing situation in the realm of happenings concerning social justice. This would certainly be a step in the right direction and would contribute in not only highlighting the powers of parliament but also bring about much needed and desired awareness among the implementing agencies and general public alike.

Another important initiative by the Hon. Speaker, Lok Sabha, Shri Somnath Chatterjee was the Inaugural Professor Hiren Mukerjee Memorail Parliamentary Lecture, which was delivered by Prof. Amartya Sen on 11th August, 2008. The theme of the First Lecture was 'The Demands of Social Justice'. Prof. Sen reminded of the speech of Hiren Mukerjee about the need for a social commitment to help produce a society that "enables all people to rise to the full stature of their being." Hon. Speaker introduced this Lecture Series with a view to help bring in some of the issues of great concern to the common people of our country and of contemporary relevance to the centre-stage of our socio-political discourse. He thought it right to think that it is only appropriate that the Parliament, being the highest representative body of the people, should initiate that process. In his welcome address, he stated, "we have to go a long way in building a progressive and prosperous India that our Founding Fathers had visualized for the country at the dawn of Independence. Providing social and economic justice to the vast segments of the masses who have been kept out of the mainstream of our socio-political life should be among the core concerns of our country today....." He is sure that this Lecture would stimulate a national debate on the need to create conditions for all our citizens, regardless of their caste and creed; to enjoy justice and equality; and other democratic rights for a dignified existence.

11th Five Year Plan (2007-12)

In his foreword to the Eleventh Five Year Plan (2007-12) – Inclusive Growth, Vol. 1, Prime Minister laid emphasis on the need to ensure that growth is widely spread so that its benefits, in terms of income and employment, are adequately shared by the poor and weaker sections of our society, especially the Scheduled Castes (SCs) and the Scheduled Tribes (STs), Other Backward Classes (OBCs) and minorities. If this has to be turned into reality, the further stated, "the growth must be inclusive in the broadest term. It must occur not just in our major cities but also in our villages and small towns."

Volume 6 of the Eleventh Five Year Plan document deals with Social Justice. It deals with the Scheduled Castes (SCs) and the Scheduled Tribes (STs), Other Backward Classes (OBCs) and Minorities. Apart from them, persons with disabilities (orthopaedic, visual, hearing, speech and mental disabilities), older persons, victims of substance and alcohol abuse, street children, beggars and victims of substances, who have been discussed in 'Other Vulnerable Groups'.

Government has been making efforts to ensure overall development of 'Other Vulnerable Groups' of the society in multifarious ways. Its main target is to improve educational development, economic development, ensuring protective measures, providing access to income earning assets in the field of agricultural land and capital assets, improving their employment situation, economic status, improving their representation in government services, ensuring their reservation in education and employment, ensuing affordable and accountable primary health care facilities, preventing land alienation, ensuring their social development, etc.

In the 11th Plan, a tentative outlay of Rs.13,043 crore has been earmarked for the Ministry of Social Justice and Empowerment for the development of SCs, OBs and other vulnerable groups.[9] Period review of schemes, plans, programmes and programmes should be carried out from time to time if we really want to see the success stories. Initiatives should be undertaken to ensure that these funds are spent and SCs, OBs and other vulnerable groups get the benefits of its successful implementation. Enough funds should be allocated for undertaking research on the whole gamut of issues relating to Disabled Persons and Other Vulnerable Groups. Above all, monitoring and evaluation mechanism should be in place at every stage to ensure that Disabled persons and other vulnerable groups derive benefits of such schemes of the Government.

Parliament, Press and Social Justice

Parliament's role in delivering the social justice is tremendous. The role of the Press in bringing more issues relating to rendering social justice before the people would create a conducive atmosphere. Parliament can be made more vibrant by bringing before it more issues. Coverage of parliament in press should be increased to a very great extent. Press should also keep in mind the efforts of the MPs to bring issues concerning social justice on the floor of both Houses of Parliament. At present, it is not so. This trend should be corrected forthwith.

Similarly, parliament should generate public awareness about its role, powers and functioning, particularly matters concerning social justice.

Parliament wields enormous power in the governance of the country. The actions of government can be questioned and scrutinized by Parliament in its functioning. This advantage should be taken seriously by bringing more and more issues concerning social justice.

If one is an avid follower of parliamentary debates, one can easily decipher how press plays a role in almost every aspect of the debate. Members keep churning out comments, figures, and the performance of the programmes of the government debate after debate, day after day. It was rightly stated that: "Most of the raw materials, for parliamentary questions, motions, debates and discussions, comes from the daily press and this is an important instrument on which a Member relies."[10]

There cannot be two opinions on the fact that the exposure given by the press to the parliamentary news and debates, to say the least, is minimal. This sorry state of affairs can be altered by highlighting many issues and debates that take place in Parliament during the Sessions and take the parliamentary news and parliamentary debates many notches up in standard. Press can make general public and readers more aware of the decisions and debates that take place in Parliament during the Sessions. Parliamentary debates should be given more prominence in newspapers, which would attract the attention of readers of newspapers, and would ultimately help the public to form an opinion on important issues discussed in Parliament. By this way, Press can awake public awareness on important national issues, which would result in more vibrant democracy and nation building in the long run.

We can revitalize Parliament's contribution to democracy and nation building with the help of national press. Public opinion is formed on many issues with the help of press. There is a general opinion that press is an extension of parliament. No doubt, press plays a very significant and vital role in highlighting what is transpiring in Parliament by giving wide publicity about the matters taken up and discussed in Parliament. But this is limited only during the period when Parliament is in Sessions. Parliamentary debates should be given more prominence in the newspapers, which would ultimately help the public to form an opinion on as important an issue like taking care of the Disabled Persons in every walk of life. By this way, Press can awake public awareness on important national issues, which would result in more vibrant democracy and nation building in the long run.

Ensuring effectiveness of Acts is a Herculean task to the Government. But if taken seriously, it would go a long way in dispensing social justice to the poor and needy of the country. Print and electronic media play a significant role here in delivering social justice to the people in this vast country.

Radio and Television plays an important role in take the programmes of the government to the disadvantaged sections of the society. Government implements various schemes and programmes for the welfare of Scheduled Castes, Other Backward Classes, etc. These programmes create awareness about the schemes and programmes among the target groups. Print Media too plays its part when it advertises the schemes and programmes of the Ministry on the important events of national and international significance such as Dr. B.R. Ambedkar Birthday on 6th December, International Day of Persons with Disabilities on 3rd December, International Day of Older Persons on 1st October, International Day against Drug Abuse and Illicit Trafficking on 26th June, etc.

Exhibitions by the Government too contribute to the awareness of the programmes and schemes of the Ministry. It reaches out to the general public and those who are in need of it. Ministry participates in the India International Trade Fair in New Delhi, Dilli Haat, New Delhi, Suraj Kund Mela in Haryana, etc.

Conclusion – Influence of Parliament

Strenuous efforts should be made by the Government to make Parliament more effective in ensuring that social justice is offered to people who deserve the most. It would not be out of place to say here that Parliament should convene a brainstorming session on how to enforce the laws for bringing about social justice in all spheres of society and in the implementation of various plans, schemes, and programmes that are meant for enforcing social justice in the country.

Lok Sabha Television, a brainchild of the current Lok Sabha Speaker, Hon'ble Somnath Chatterjee, came into being during the 14th Lok Sabha. The primary intention for the introduction of Lok Sabha Television was faithful reporting about whatever transpires in the Chamber of Lok Sabha. In his address at the valedictory session of the 14th All India Whips Conference, Mumbai on 5 February, 2008, Speaker, Lok Sabha remarked: "It was felt that for strengthening Parliamentary democracy it is essential that the people of the country at large, who have constituted the Lok Sabha by electing their representatives as Members, should have the right to know what was happening inside the House, how the Members were behaving, what laws were passed, what issues were discussed, amongst other things."[11] One of the main reasons for the introduction of Lok Sabha Television is that people who come to witness the proceedings from the Visitor's Gallery face a lot of inconvenience. With the introduction of Lok Sabha Television, the whole country can watch the proceedings of Lok Sabha. In order words, Parliament has now reached every TV-owning or watching citizen of India and the ties of every India have been cemented with the wonderful building called Parliament of India. More and more programmes, debates and discussions should be aired to reach out to the disadvantaged people and to bring awareness about the programmes, schemes and policies of the Government for their upliftment.

Programmes and films aimed at sensitizing and highlighting the struggles and problems being faced on a day to day basis by the Disabled Persons in the prime time would have an indelible impact and would go a log way in making government and private institutions disabled-friendly.

Parliament's main function is to legislate. Presently, due to coalition politics, Parliament is not able to contribute adequately in this sphere. Government has to take all its coalition partners with it if it wants to implement any scheme or programme. In the process, it faces many hurdles. Hence, avenues for revitalizing Parliament's contribution to democracy and nation building are far and wide. Certainly, Parliament and parliamentary debates can be made more vibrant by merely bringing before Parliament more important concerns of different facts of social justice for discussion and for finding discernible solutions. Parliament's time can be used in a meaningful manner to highlight peoples' issues or concerns of downtrodden people and having threadbare discussions on issues involving education, health, housing and other needs of the Schedule Castes, Disabled, Aged Persons, etc. More participation of Members in Parliamentary debates would bring out the finer elements of issues having impact on people.

Efforts are underway through the implementation of mega project to make Government schools in Delhi disabled-friendly.[12] It is reported that a sum of Rs.245 crore is allocated for upgrading the 198 schools to make them disabled-friendly. Special teachers have been appointed and hearing aids and spectacles are also provided to the children with special needs. Apart from the above, 50 Special Educators had been recruited; 1,048 visually impaired students in Government schools of Delhi and aided schools had been given 80 per cent of the text books in Braille.[13]

Before serious initiative is taken to discuss the issue of social justice to disabled persons, we have to remove the gross injustice meted out to them. A conducive atmosphere should be created for the disabled person to lead a normal life. It is certainly a welcome feature to see in the recent past buildings are designed to make them disabled persons-friendly. Central and State Governments and other actors concerned with 'disabled persons' should address the problems being faced by them and ensure that they contribute productively in the development process of the country. To achieve this Herculean task, proper and effective implementation of various acts concerning social justice, in general, and addressing the struggles being faced by persons with disabilities (orthopaedic, visual, hearing, speech and mental disabilities), older persons, victims of substance and alcohol abuse, street children, beggars and victims of substances, who have been discussed under the heading 'Other Vulnerable Groups' in Chapter 6 of the 11th Plan. A national debate is required on the nuances of 'disability'. As discussed in this topic, many steps have been undertaken by the governments since Independence but much more is expected if we have to satisfy them. Special efforts and drive should be initiated by the Government to ensure that social justice is meted out to the Disabled Persons and 'Other Vulnerable Groups of the society' so that they could become part of the mainstream.

REFERENCES

1. http://socialjustice.nic.in/aboutdivision3.html, retrieved on 13.07.2009.
2. Social Justice (In Indian Perspective) by D.R. Jatava, p.124.
3. http://socialjustice.nic.in/aboutdivision3.html, retrieved on 13.07.2009.
4. http://socialjustice.nic.in/faq.html, retrieved on 13.07.2009.
5. Cells on Parliamentary Forum, http://164.100.24.209/newls/cells%20on%20parforam.htm Assessed on 3.4.2008.
6. Ibid.
7. Ibid.
8. http://164.100.24.209/newls/bureau/bpstAims.htm Assessed on 3.4.2008.
9. Eleventh Five Year Plan Document, Planning Commission, New Delhi, 2007.
10. Ibid. p. 77.
11. http://speakerloksabha.nic.in Assessed on 3.4.2008.
12. Parvaiz Sultan, "Mega project underway to make Government schools disabled-friendly", *Pioneer* (New Delhi), 16 November, 2008
13. Ibid.

PART IV

GENDERED DIMENSION

12

Disability, Poverty and Sustainable Development: A Gendered Perspective

Amit Rahul and Rashmi Sinha

Introduction

The disability is recognized as one of the several factors, such as, gender, age and caste, which interact to impoverish people and keep them poor. It is understood here as a complex system of social restrictions imposed on people with impairments resulting in a denial of rights and equal opportunities which leads to the perpetuation of poverty among them. Poverty should not be simply understood here as the consequence of the lack of resources. Some people are unable to access existing resources because of who they are, what they believe or where they live. Such discrimination is a form of exclusion and a cause of poverty.[1] Because disability and poverty are inextricably linked, poverty can never be eradicated until disabled people enjoy equal rights with non-disabled people.[2]

The disabled people are so severely excluded from all areas of society that there is not even comparable or reliable data on incidence, distribution and trends of disability, let alone the extent of disabled people's poverty. Despite this lack of comparable data there is plenty of anecdotal and more substantiated evidence to show that disabled people are generally amongst the poorest of the poor. It is already known that living in poverty increases the likelihood of getting impairment. The studies have also shown that the disabled people generally experience higher rates of poverty as a result of being disabled and that when people living in poverty become disabled they are often more severely marginalized than the wealthier people.[3]

There are several glaring constraints that prevent the disabled persons from enjoying equal opportunities. The lack of awareness of the rights and needs of disabled persons by society in general, lack of education, medical care, rehabilitation services and support services, skills training and employment are some of the biggest constraints. The question of the awareness of the human rights of disabled persons by society as a whole also plays an important role. All of these contribute to the perpetuation of poverty, deprivation and marginalization of the disabled. From the economic viewpoint, one can infer that poverty and disablement are synonymous with each other.

The reduction of poverty in its many dimensions is one of the overarching goals of the sustainable development paradigm. The sustainable development implies a broad view of human welfare, a long-term perspective about the consequences of today's activities, and the full involvement of civil society to reach viable solutions. The concept of sustainability means many different things to different people, and a large part of humanity around the world still live without access to basic necessities. The theory of sustainable development goes to the heart of tackling a number of inter-related global issues, such as, poverty, inequality, hunger and environmental degradation. The idea of sustainable development grew from numerous environmental movements in earlier decades and was defined in 1987 by the World Commission on Environment and Development as the "Development that meets the needs of the present without compromising the ability of future generations to meet their own needs".[4] The primary objective of the sustainable development is to reduce the absolute poverty of the world's poor by providing lasting and secure livelihoods that minimize resource depletion, environmental degradation, cultural disruption and social instability.

Today the term has got broader in meaning and is applied equally to the shared and inter-linked responsibilities of environmental protection and human development. Sustainable development can only be achieved through long-term investments in economics, environmental and human capital. At present, the female half of the world's human capital is undervalued and under-utilized the world over. Better use of the world's female population could increase economic growth, reduce poverty, enhance societal well-being and help ensure sustainable development in all countries. Closing the gender gap depends on enlightened government policies which take gender dimensions into account. And for this, taking care of the needs of the most marginalized and vulnerable section among the women, particularly the disabled women should constitute the most important agenda of any sustainable development framework. Situating disability and poverty in the realm of sustainable development paradigm will give a new dimension to the whole concept of sustainable development.

The people with disabilities are particularly vulnerable to poverty and exclusion. The disabled people are disproportionately poor, and poverty, in turn, creates disabling living conditions. Often 'poverty' is synonymous with low income but increasingly the multi-dimensionality of poverty has come into focus within the development literature. Amartya Sen identifies four dimensions of poverty such as opportunity (access to markets and employment); capability (access to health and education); security (vulnerability to economic risks and to all forms of violence); and empowerment (power within and beyond the household).[5] The disabled women have to face a majority of these poverty situations. The women with disabilities are one of the most marginalized groups - both in the women's movement and within the disability rights movement itself. Under the circumstances their vulnerability and isolation increases manifold.

The studies have shown that disability is very intricately linked with the issue of poverty.[6] It is both a cause and consequence of poverty.[7] The overall goal of weeding out poverty and ensuring sustainable development cannot be realized unless the rights and needs of people with disabilities in general and disabled women in particular are taken into account. The United Nations data on disability shows that one in 20 persons has a disability.[8] A considerable number of the disabled lives in the third world countries which are harnessing their potential to come up at par with the developed nations of the world.[9] According to the UN estimates, more than three out of four of the world's disabled live in the developing countries. The estimates and studies have shown that more often than not they are among the poorest of the poor.[10]

Disability is limiting and does not allow a person to utilize his or her full potential.[11] The debilitating limits of disability could be seen in the access to education, employment and social acceptability. This leads to economic and social exclusion. The poor people with disabilities are caught in a vicious cycle of poverty and disability, each being both a cause and a consequence of the other. Although, disability and poverty affect men and women worldwide, the subordinate status and situation of women in the society further increases their vulnerability and exclusion. Both poverty and disability affect an individual's capability, especially women, impacting their participation in society.

The problem of disability gets all the more compounded when the disabled happens to be a woman.[12] The disabled women have to face double discrimination, both for being woman and for being disabled, although, the social status of disabled women might vary according to individual circumstances and to the community in which they live. The evidences have shown that similar nature of disability for women and men may lead to two different ways of treatment being meted by the family of the disabled person and the larger society. While, women are forced to stay indoors and pass their time without not much provision for education and social interaction, men are allowed and even encouraged to go for education and look for 'out-of home' job if the level of disability so allows.

The general attitude of the society towards disabled women is that they will not prove to be good wife or mothers. The recent example where the Supreme Court had to intervene to ensure that a mentally unstable woman was allowed to give birth to her child, which her family was opposed to, shows the apathetic nature of the family and society towards disabled women. Disability, whether mental or physical, does not disable a person but, discrimination, marginalization, social stigma and poverty does. Social apathy marginalizes persons with disabilities and prevents them from fully participating in society they live. Today, we have data on the socio-economic status of the marginalized and vulnerable groups such as scheduled castes, scheduled tribes, women, etc, however, the lack of a comprehensive data base of information on the extent of poverty of disabled persons, the most marginalized and vulnerable among such groups, emphasizes their marginalized and invisible status.

A woman's main role, in most communities, is still to be a wife, mother, and homemaker while the man is the main decision-maker and income earner. Since education and vocational training are seen as investments for higher-value employment, a woman is less likely to have the opportunity to receive them. While public attitudes are changing, illiteracy rates among women worldwide are falling, and more and more women are entering into the labour market, the situation has changed little for women with disabilities. When women with disabilities do not have access to resources, education, and other opportunities, they are more vulnerable to poverty, exploitation, and abuse. Without confidence in and awareness of their rights, they are often socially marginalized.[13] The plight of the women with disability is very movingly highlighted in the short verse presented below:

People don't see me
They think I'm useless
Say any word they want.
Don't I think as they do?
I need to be recognized!

If I walk down the street
They say: "There's a cripple!"
If I handle my crutches
They move away quickly
As though a plane's taking off.

Don't do anything for me!
I need to be on my own.

If I go for work
They say, "No - give her this special, light job."
But "special" means "discrimination".

I need to express my rights
To say what I want.
And remember
My choice is not a mistake.
Don't be shy for me. Let me be shy for myself.
Let me speak for myself.[14]

This paper assesses the significance of disabled women as a key sustainable development issue, and its importance in relation to poverty and human rights. It also sets out ways in which the paradigm of sustainable development can help incorporate the rights and needs of women with disabilities into the mainstream of poverty reduction work and the achievement of human rights. This paper will examine the economic and social impact of being women and disabled. The question, of who determines what and for whom varies from group to group, but is always based on the 'balance or imbalance of power'. This is a form of social oppression that stems from systemic problems rooted in the present social and political system.

Triple Oppression: Being Woman, Poor and Disabled

Despite their significant numbers, women and girls with disabilities remain hidden and silent, their concerns unknown and their rights overlooked. Throughout the society, in urban and rural communities alike, disabled women have to face triple discrimination by society. Not only because of their disabilities, but also because they are female and poor. In many countries, especially developing ones, there is a feminization of poverty in relation to women with disabilities, who are marginalized within an already marginalized group; of women in poverty, those with disabilities are frequently the poorest.[15] Most women with disabilities are more likely to be extremely poor, have little or no schooling, be without vocational skills, be unemployed, have less access to public services, be unmarried or childless and be physically, sexually, or psychologically abused.

They make up, without doubt, one of the most excluded and isolated groups of people in every society, being triply disadvantaged by their disabilities, by their sex, and by poverty.

Like all other disabled people, women with disabilities are often treated as if their particular disability has affected all their other abilities. In society's eyes they are not capable of earning an income, let alone of living independently.[16] While with education, government legislation, increasing awareness and opportunities the conditions are improving for the normal women, but the situation remains largely unchanged for the women with disabilities. The general attitude is still that a disabled woman has little hope of becoming a wife or a mother, or of getting a real job. She therefore is a burden to her family or the state – a dependant for the rest of her life. Women and girls with disabilities face double jeopardy through their status as women and as a person with disabilities. They continue to be excluded from access to health care, social protection schemes, education, employment and enjoyment of all human rights.

The exclusion of women with disabilities occurs at different levels—the planning process, lack of funds for accommodations, their absence in the women's agenda, and omissions in research, action, policy and services designed to assist women in overcoming discrimination. The women with disabilities face many barriers in realizing their potential. From childhood, many of them are deprived of their self-determination, become victims of domestic violence, sexual abuse in institution and work place. They are denied of family life. Until not so long ago, it was not so uncommon to hear of forced sterilization of them, and not given any reproductive care.[17] Maternal rights of disabled women have been denied due to their disability. Because of disability, many women cannot get job even when they are qualified. There are few representatives of women with disabilities both in women's organizations and disabled people's organizations. Certain cultural practices might increase the risk of causing disabilities in women.[18] The extent and nature of marginalization, deprivation, exclusion and peripheral treatment meted out to the women faced with disability has been examined around the following factors:

Attitudes: Isolation and Invisibility

Strong stereotyped and negative attitudes towards disabled people are still found in our society. The women are generally discriminated against due to gender bias but disabled women face compound discrimination by being both women and disabled. Much of the discrimination experienced by disabled women is based on an implicit notion that they are not the same as other women and so cannot be expected to share the same rights and aspirations. The isolation and confinement based on culture and traditions, attitudes and prejudices often affect disabled women more than men. This isolation of disabled women leads to low self-esteem and negative feelings. Lack of appropriate support services and lack of adequate education result in low economic status, which, in turn, creates dependency on families or care-givers.

Some societies go so far as to assign fault to a mother who gives birth to a disabled child, especially so if the mother is a disabled woman. The disabled women and men can experience different kinds of attitudes based on gender discrimination. While men are still seen as the major bread-winners and leaders of society, a disabled man, considered 'less of a man', won't conform to that stereotype. Similarly, a disabled woman won't conform to the feminine stereotype of wife, partner or mother and some lose the right to keep their children. The culture plays a big part in reducing disabled women's role in social, parental and economic life. Because disabled people are often excluded from society, the attitudes of the public are heavily influenced by how disabled people are portrayed in the media. The disabled women are seldom seen in ordinary roles as worker or mother.

Education

Literacy and a basic education are essential for enabling the poor to access the benefits offered by development initiatives and market opportunities. Basic education is therefore a precondition for sustainable development. The children with disabilities have very limited access to education. Only 1-2 percent of children with disabilities in developing countries receive a formal education.[19]

Considering the importance of education for the all round development of the human personality and its role in bettering the life chances of the person the lack of universal and inclusive education might lead to the perpetuation of poverty and social exclusion.[20] The problem is severe in the case of the girl child who has to bear with the still continuing oppressive patriarchal order in our society and all the more grotesque for the disabled female child who is thought of as a burden on the family and the society. The literature on disabled girls and education is sparse. This holds true for countries at all levels of development.[21]

The available data, focusing on literacy, indicate that women and girls with disabilities fare less well in the educational arena than either their disabled male or non-disabled female counterparts. For example, UNESCO, the World Blind Union and others estimate the literacy rate for disabled women as one percent, compared to an estimate of about three percent for people with disabilities as a whole.[22] The avowed goal of providing education for all cannot be achieved as long as children with disabilities are left out of schools. If we take the access to school as an indicator of the gendered bias towards the disabled we can look at the enrolment ratio and drop-out rate for the boys and girls facing disability. The studies have shown that the boys with disabilities attend school more frequently than girls with disabilities. Therefore, the needs of girls with disabilities may be more special than needs of any other groups and have to be addressed in all spheres of education.

Health Care

Human health in its broadest sense of physical, mental and spiritual wellbeing is to a great extent dependent on the access of the citizen to a healthy environment. For a healthy, productive and fulfilling life every individual should have the physical and economic access to a balanced diet, safe drinking water, clean air, sanitation, environmental hygiene, primary health care and education. Like most women, women with disabilities often find it difficult to get the health care they need. Disabled women find barriers to care when health facilities do not have ramps for wheelchair users, do not have information in Braille or on audio cassettes for vision-impaired people, do not have sign language interpreters for women who are deaf, and do not have people who can assist women who have trouble learning or understanding. Another problem is that doctors and other health workers are not usually trained to understand the health needs disabled women may have.

The maternal health care is often denied to disabled women, either because it is not considered right for them to bear children, or because the available services do not consider their particular needs. The basic health and educational facilities in developing countries need to be strengthened. People should be empowered through education and awareness to participate in managing preventive health care related to environmental sanitation and hygiene. Studies on the quality of health care services available to disabled women are rare. Around two third disabled women in the world live in developing countries. In many of these countries women are at a much higher risk to become disabled because of malnutrition due to male preference. Because of male preference, disabled women receive less immunization and are less often taken to the doctor. Because of gender discrimination women with disabilities receive only 1/5th of the world's rehabilitation services.[23]

The health care facilities are often inaccessible to women in wheelchairs, women who are deaf or blind and women with intellectual disabilities. Why don't women with disabilities have access to appropriate health care services? It's because of barriers which take many forms. Most health care facilities are not accessible because of architectural or communicative barriers. The health care facilities should meet the requirements of the disabled persons and necessary steps should be taken in this regard so as to make the health services disabled friendly. We believe they do not open their doors to disabled persons because disabled persons are not the desired patients. They often don't fit into the profitability quotient and materialistic expectations of the majority of the health care providers.

Many doctors and health practitioners, frankly, refuse to treat disabled persons. Often doctors have no respect for disabled women's right to privacy. As a result many women with disabilities who live independently choose not to see a doctor at all. This in turn contributes to the lack of health services due to architectural and other barriers. Disabled women need to be protected against both forms of human rights violations regarding their right to health: disabled women need access to health care and the health care services need to be respectful and non-discriminating. Governments bear the ultimate responsibility that doctors and other health care providers begin to respect the human rights of disabled women.

Government Policies

It should be noted that disability as an issue has never been included in any political agenda although disabled persons too have the right to vote. Although, a series of efforts have been made by the government and other organizations to improve the conditions of the disabled people and bring them into the mainstream there is a long way to go before the 'differently-abled' can finally come into their own. Moreover, the altruistic paradigm is reflected in governmental policies, which until very recently looked at disability as a welfare issue. Even now, most government efforts are targeted at strengthening non-governmental organizations without making any direct interventions.[24] Also, the disability legislation adopts a gendered approach, with the result that out of twenty-eight chapters outlining various issues, not a single one addresses the problems of disabled women.[25] There is a need for the government to make necessary steps both to prevent disability and to ensure the inclusion of persons with disabilities in their programmes.

The consideration of the rights and needs of persons with disabilities, together with the prevention of the causes of disabilities, is essential if the overall aim of the sustainable development is to be realized. The World Bank has determined that it is impossible to achieve the international Millennium Development Goals (MDGs) if disability issues and people with disabilities are not included. Reaching all round development will not be possible unless disabled people are brought into the equation. As James Wolfensohn, former president of the World Bank put it, "disabled people are also more likely than other people to live in grinding poverty and the disabled in their countries live at the bottom of the pile".[26] The disabled people and more particularly the disabled women have always been accorded step-motherly treatment in any government policy and planning. If development programs are to succeed in reducing poverty and strengthening good governance, then they need to more pro-actively involve and include persons with disabilities.

Physical and Sexual Abuse

The women with disabilities are two to three times more likely to be victims of physical and sexual abuse than non-disabled women.[27] Their access to reproductive health care is minimal and as a result they suffer greater vulnerability to reproductive health problems and sexually transmitted diseases. The women with disabilities have to struggle and confront vulnerabilities in their own efforts to end sexual abuse. These include frequent lack of privacy, the physical difficulties associated with escaping sexual abuse, and higher rates of exposure to institutional facilities where mistreatment is notoriously rampant and thus normalized.[28]

There is a greater reliance of women with disabilities on others for care and this makes them increasingly vulnerable to physical and mental abuse. They fear that reporting abusive providers and companions might trigger the end of a relationship and loss of essential care. Even in healthcare, there is a lack of awareness regarding women with disabilities and reproductive health care needs. More often than not, it is assumed that they do not form part of the target groups because being disabled is associated with being sexless or asexual. Many parents of young girls with disabilities are often advised to remove the uterus of their wards for safety reasons.

Employment

Even though disabled people constitute a significant 5 to 6 percent of the population of India, their needs for employment remain unsatisfied, in spite of the implementation of the Persons with Disabilities Act, 1995, which reserves 3 per cent of all categories of jobs in the Government sector for disabled persons.[29] The negative attitude that most employers have towards the disabled is also a significant barrier to their mainstreaming. The problem is all the more glaring for the disabled women who are not usually part of employment debates and initiatives. They are usually at least twice as unlikely as disabled men to get a job.[30] Excluded from opportunities, disabled women are on the whole desperately poor. While poverty is a result of discrimination, it is also a cause of further discrimination. As has been discussed earlier that poverty is not only the lack of money but of resources, skills, knowledge, and social connections. Without those resources, disabled women have very limited access to institutions, services, markets, and employment.

The extensive discrimination against women with disabilities violates the principle of equality of rights and their human dignity. They are denied equal opportunities in social, economic, and political life. The especially difficult situation of women with disabilities has been recognized nationally and internationally. However, there is as yet not enough action or results, at least to the extent that women with disabilities everywhere are able to experience a tangible improvement in their lives. Where disabled women have been given opportunities for training and work, they have shown that they can be loyal and reliable workers. They are highly motivated because, while for most people work is a means of gaining financial independence, for women with disabilities having a job also means becoming part of society – something others take for granted.[31]

The Need to Integrate Disability in Sustainable Development Theory

The eradication of poverty is the greatest challenge facing the world toady and therefore any sustainable development effort would be incomplete without addressing this issue. The very process of integrating disability in general and women's disability in particular as a category of analysis and system of representation deepens, expands and challenges sustainable development theory. The incorporation of disability and disabled will surely lead to the broadening of the range of the sustainable development theory and make it more representative, egalitarian and wider in scope and reach. Any sustainable development mechanism should try to address the issues of education, employment vocational training and social inclusion of the disabled women in order to break the vicious circle of neglect, isolation, and poverty of such women faced with disability.

Unless disabled people are brought into the sustainable development framework it will be impossible to make development truly inclusive. The sustainable development approach should also see to it that that the disabled people have the chance to take command of their own lives, rather than be passive recipients of care or charity. The inclusion of the rights-based approach to development which has been increasingly adopted by the government and international development agencies throughout the world will increase the relevance, applicability and reach of the sustainable development approach. It is clear that unless disability is included in the sustainable development framework, the prospects for achieving the goal of securing the development for all will be substantially diminished.

Equalization of opportunities should be made a basic concept in the principle of sustainable development. Through this process the various systems of society and the environment such as services, information, and documentation should be made available to all – particularly to those who are excluded by social, economic, cultural, and political barriers. It is only through universal access that the all round and sustainable development of the disabled is possible. Access in its fullest sense refers to physical access, communication access, and social access to facilities, services, training, and jobs. Physical access means that people with disabilities can, without assistance, approach, enter, pass to and from, and make use of an area and its facilities without undue difficulties.

Conclusion

It is the aspiration of every disabled woman – to be able to have friends, to go to school, to have the qualifications and skills for a good job and then do the job well, to be independent, to be respected, to give and receive love. In other words, they want to have a life like other men and women. There is an urgent need to counter the belief that a disabled person is an object of pity who always needs assistance from somebody else. Though, the government has framed policies and laws like the National Policy for Persons with Disability, 2005 and the Persons with Disabilities Act, 1995 and has launched schemes for the general upliftment of the disabled and to improve their living conditions, the efforts are far from satisfactory and much more needs to be done in this regard. Also, merely striving for the general improvements in living conditions will not be enough.

Poverty, disability and gender affect an individual's capability, impacting their full participation in society. Bringing the disabled women into the purview of sustainable development theory is crucial for the all inclusive developmental efforts. Specific steps are still required, not only for prevention, but also to ensure that people with disabilities (more so for women) are able to participate fully in the development process, obtain a fair share of the benefits, and claim their rights as full and equal members of society. To increase the visibility of disabled women it is the responsibility of the state to include them in any sustainable development paradigm and ensure that the plans and programmes are gender sensitive. The women with disabilities should be included in any decision making process concerning them. A major thrust at the policy level is necessary to ensure equity and justice for them.

The sustainable development approach if applied with complete sincerity and dedication and accountability would ensure that the most marginalized, deprived and often forgotten section of our population are brought into the mainstream. The disability in general is seen by planners and policy makers as welfare rather than developmental and rightful, or as peripheral rather than central to the development process. For the all round inclusive development process which is the most important requirement of the sustainable development framework it should be made sure that disabled in general and women in particular are provided equal opportunities to excel in their desired field and do not continue to remain at the periphery of the society.

REFERENCES

1. DFID, "Realizing Human Rights for Poor People: Strategies for Achieving the International Development Targets", 2000.
2. Lee, Helen, Discussion Paper for Oxfam: Disability as a Development Issue and how to Integrate a Disability Perspective into the SCO. Oxford: Oxfam, 1999.
3. Rebecca Yeo, "Chronic Poverty and Disability", Action on Disability

and Development (ADD) Background Paper Number 4, Chronic Poverty Research Centre, August 2001.

4. Anup Shah, "Sustainable Development Introduction", 2005, Last checked by the author on 17th August, 2009. http://www. global issues.org/article/408/sustainable-development-introduction
5. Sen, Amartya, "Development as Freedom. Oxford University Press: Oxford, UK, 2001.
6. Peat, M, "Disability in the Developing World", in M.A. McColl and J.E. Bickenbach (ed), *Introduction to Disability and Handicap,* W.B Saunders, Canada, 1998, pp. 43-53.
7. Elwan, A., "Poverty and Disability: A Survey of the Literature", Social Protection Discussion Paper No. 9932, World Bank, Washington D.C.
8. DFID, "Disability, Poverty and Development", February, 2000.
9. E.Helander, "Prejudice and Dignity: An Introduction to Community Based Rehabilitation", UNDP, 1992.
10. Patricia Welch, "Applying the Capability approach in Examining Disability, Poverty and Gender", Conference Proceedings-Promoting Women's Capability: Examining Nussbaum's Capability approaches, Von Hugel Institute, St Edmunds College, Cambridge, 9-10 September, 2002.
11. Aberley, P., "Work, Utopia and Impairment", in Barton, L, (ed), Disability and Society: Emerging Issues and Rights, Longman, London, 1996.
12. Patricia Welch, op.cit, 9-10 September, 2002, p.2.
13. Jane Maxwell, Julia Watts Belser and Darlena David, "Understanding Women with Disabilities", Hesperian Foundation, 2007.
14. "People Don't See Me" - by Estella Jossum, Independent Living Institute, "Disabled Women", Published by Disability Awareness in Action, London, United Kingdom, 1996.
15. Charlotte McClain, "Women with Disabilities: From Invisible to Visible Citizens", Meeting of the Ad Hoc Committee, 16-27 June 2003: NGO Bulletins: Disability Negotiations Bulletin, Vol. 2, No. 9, June 26, 2003.
16. Foo Gaik Sim, "Integrating Women and Girls with Disabilities into Mainstream Vocational Training", ILO Publication, Bangkok, 1999.
17. ESCAP, UN, "Women with Disabilities," Asia-Pacific NGO Forum, Beijing, 2004.
18. ESCAP, UN, Task Force on Women with Disabilities Thematic Working Group on Disability and related concerns (TWG-DC), Beijing, September, 2004.

19. See, http://info.stakes.fi/ssd/EN/disabilityandpoverty/guidelines/themes/index.htm
20. http://siteresources.worldbank.org/EDUCATION/Resources/Education-Notes/EdNotesDisability.pdf. The World Bank Education Note characterizes inclusive education as follows: "Inclusive Education means that schools and teachers accommodate and respond to individual learners; this inclusiveness itself benefits the school, the teachers and all students."
21. Rousso, H. "Strong Proud Sisters: Girls and Young Women with Disabilities", Washington, DC: Center for Women Policy Studies, 2001.
22. Groce, N. "Women with Disabilities in the Developing World. *Journal of Disability Policy Studies*. 8, 1&2, 1997, pp. 178-192.
23. Theresia Degener, "Disabled Women and the Right to Health Care", Presented at Hunter College, June 7th, 2000, New York.
24. Anita Ghai, "Disabled women: An Excluded agenda of Indian feminism", *Hypatia*, Vol. 17, No. 3, Feminism and Disability, Part 2, Summer, 2002, pp. 49-66.
25. Anita Ghai, op.cit, 2002, p. 53.
26. Disability-Key to tackling Poverty, http://www.developments.org.uk/article
27. http://www.azrapeprevention.org/summaries/disabled.html
28. Family Violence Against Women with Disabilities, http://dawn.thot.net/violence_wwd.html
29. Anita Ghai, op.cit, 2002.
30. Independent Living Institute, "Disabled Women", Published by Disability Awareness in Action, London, 1996.
31. Foo Gaik Sim, "Integrating Women and Girls with Disabilities into Mainstream Vocational Training", op.cit, p. 2.

13

Disabled Women in Search of their Identity: Himachal in Focus

Ruchi Ramesh

Twenty five hundred years ago, when young Gautam Buddha left his princely home in the foothills of the Himalayas in search of enlightenment, he was moved specifically by the sight of morality, morbidity and disability around him and it moved him immensely. Disability is part and parcel of every society. It is not individual condition but society which disables people with impairments. It is worth mentioning at the very outset that impairment is not something difficult to overcome but it is attitude of society towards people with impairment which is difficult to surmount. The struggle for disables is not only for their survival but also for weeding out the social disability in order to bring social change. It is social disability which results in the exclusion, non-participation and discrimination of disabled people. Coleridge (1993) is of the opinion that if abled -bodied people did not react with horror, fear, anxiety, distaste, hostility or patronizing behavior towards disabled people, then there would be no problem. Disability is not so much a physical condition but as a psycho-social crisis for those afflicted. It is not so much the disability which paralyses, but handicaps caused by society.

A society itself is invisibly disabled for a critique of its inhumane norms and values. Hence the thesis 'the disables need society and society needs the disabled'. Within a social model framework, disability is redefined as social oppression experienced by people with perceived impairments become disabled people, denied the opportunities and support to take up the rights and responsibilities of full citizenship, to follow ordinary life course pathways, to enjoy ordinary life chances.

The roots of disability could be traced back to evolution of human race. At the on set of 21st century there is a fundamental gap between developed and developing nations in all parameters of resource and human security. But these prevailing imbalances of their resources could not reflect with the status of the people with disability. In majority world societies, disabled people are highly over represented among the poor and unemployed. In the West disabled people emphasis the need for equality and anti-discrimination legislation, disabled people in the developing world are still calling for their basic human survival needs to be met. The needs and priorities identified by disabled people themselves vary from those identified in developed countries. In few countries like Jordan source of income was identified as primary to their lives whereas source of income does not feature in the list of seven areas of primary needs identified by disabled people. The fact of matter is that in developed and developing countries disables are confronting with gamut of discrimination embedded with social stigmas. The meaning of disability in India is embedded in multiple cultural discourses, on the one hand disability implies to diminished capability on the other hand disability is wrath of God being punished for sin either them or their families have committed. According to International Groups of Disabled Rights "In our view, it is society which disables.... Disability is something imposed on top of our impairments, by the way we are unnecessarily isolated and excluded from full participation in society. Disabled people are therefore an oppressed group in society" (UPIAS, 1976).

Disability can strike anyone, anywhere and at any time. But it strikes often very poor, the malnutrited and less privileged. This means that women fall easy pray of disability. The women with disabilities is one of the most oppressed and marginalized groups of people in society. The women are handicapped, discriminated against merely because they are women but disability compounds this prejudice. The stigma of disability, with its myths and fears increases their social isolation. Women with disability are at high risk of being abused by society, such women are vulnerable to multiple and repeated acts of abuse or difficulty identifying the perpetrator. Additionally, it is the matter of stigmatization. Women in general have been characterized as passive, weak, naïve and dependent, these stereotypes may be more damaging to women with disabilities. National Violence Against Women Survey (NVAWS) indicates that having a severe or moderate disability places a woman at relatively greater risk of physical assault. A major Canadian study by Ridington found 40% of sample reported having been abused or raped, typically that the hands of the primary or other caregiver (Ridington, 2006). Furthermore, women with disabilities have been historically been marginalized and viewed as a socially "invisible population" due to what Warranty and Yuen referred to as "a stigmatizing social construction of disability". The stigmatization and marginalization have resulted in a historical omission of women with disabilities.

The exclusion of women with disability is not only detrimental to them but to the entire human community. The society cannot afford to continue to disregard and denigrate the role, task and services performed by women. To prevent disability in society it is of utmost importance to improve the condition of women in general and that of women with disabilities in particular. Disability creates and exacerbates poverty by increasing isolation and economic strain, not just for the individual but for the family: there is little doubt that disable people are among the poorest in poor countries. It is well recognized fact that a vicious circle is formed whereby poverty produces impairment, and impairment in a disabling society, results in poverty. To break the vicious circle of disability women as a group must be taken care of. In most of the developing countries among the major disabling conditions that women suffer are iron deficiency anaemia, chronic infectious pelvic disease, respiratory diseases, chronic malnutrition weaken the general state of health, making women more susceptible and less able to recover from illnesses.

Disable Women and Human Rights

According to capability approach of any substantive theory of ethics and political philosophy, particularly any theory of justice, has to choose an informational focus, that is, it has to decide which features of the world we should concentrate on in judging a society and in assessing justice and injustice, a person's advantage in terms of opportunities is judged to be lower than that of another if she has less capability – less real opportunity – to achieve those things that she has reason to value, obviously, the things we value most are particularly important for us to be able to achieve. The perspective does point to the central relevance of the inequality of capabilities in the assessment of social disparities, but it does not on its own, propose any specific formula for policy decisions. In judging the aggregate progress of the society, the capability approach would certainly draw attention to the huge significance of the expansion of human capabilities to all members of society. The nature of lives people can lead has been the object of attention of social analysts over the ages even though the much used economic criteria of advancement, reflected in a mass of readily produced statistics, have tended to focus specifically on the enhancement of inanimate objects of that concentration could be ultimately justified to the extent it could be only through what these objects do to the human lives they can directly or indirectly influence. The case for using instead direct indicators of the quality of life and of well being and freedom that human lives can bring has been increasingly recognized. Amartya Sen has included some specific types of rights within the category of general analysis of human Rights. There is inclusion of 'economic and social rights' which are sometimes called as 'welfare rights'. Which are seen as 'second generation' rights, such as entitlement to subsistence or to medical care. The removal of global poverty and other economic and social deprivations has thus come to centre-stage in the global engagement with human rights.

Disability is one of the most vital human concerns, Vienna Convention of international human rights in 1993 has adopted disability as one of the most crucial components and more than 150 countries of the contemporary world are signatories of this declaration. Again under the aegis of the U.N., world governments have signed on declarations which ensure the compliance of all rights to disables in 2007.

There is something very appealing in the idea that every person anywhere in the world irrespective of citizenship, residence, race, class, caste or community has some basic rights which others should respect. The message that resonates through universal declaration of Human Rights is that the quest for justice, equality, peace, security people's participation and the sustained improvements in the quality of life of every individual whether man or women are inseparable human pursuits.

A stereotypical conceptualization of people with disability as disadvantaged minority group includes the gross misperception that such individuals are less intelligent, less able to make the right decisions, less realistic, less logical, less able to determine their life than non disabled persons. Equally disconcerting is the fact that people with disabilities, particularly women, are collectively defined as social monolith. The disabled women are systematically denied the most of the human rights – the right to love, right to marriage, the right to motherhood, right to personal fulfillment. While men are more likely to marry, to enjoy the blessings of family life, in some societies it is considered somehow shocking that the disabled women should not marry. The society tends to treat women with disabilities as asexual. This has serious implication for self- esteem and self- image of disabled women (Cathy McPherson, 1991). The perceived failure to perform expected roles places extra pressure on disabled women and their families, which in turn may lead to a crisis of identity for the disabled women about their adult role, and result in social and economic problems for the whole family. The women with disabilities have in the past been excluded from the societal expectations of womanhood and motherhood particularly in the case for women with intellectual disabilities who were constituted by the eugenic movement early this century as a threat to the very structure of society because of their child bearing capacity. Consequently, many women with disabilities were subject to sterilization, constant surveillance institutionalization to prevent them from becoming mothers. The dominant discourse historically has placed them as women who are unfit to have children or to be mothers. The ethnographic studies from Iceland and Australia concluded that even those women who have strong desire for children are forced for sterilization by their families. The studies reveal that none of the women who had been involved in decision about having children, or the desire to have them, had found the processes easy or simple. The women with disability were trapped between two opposing discourses: one which focused on their own perceived desire and right to bear a child and to be a mother, and the other which has excluded them from the possibility of motherhood. Some women had internalized the societal discourse and did not see child bearing as a possibility for them.

In developing countries the situation of common development has remained pathetic due to variety of reasons. Majority of developing countries have emerged independent after the Second World War. Many among them have adopted democracy as the way of governance. Democracy insists on the common developed with special development to the marginalized. By all cannons of social justice, the disability includes as one of the worst group within marginalized groups. The component of human rights has emerged as one of the most publicized agenda of the international system with the end of the cold war. Human rights and democracy however are dependent on each other. But even in democracies, which are morally compelled to implement the egalitarian agenda of human rights, have kept mum on the compliance of these cardinal principles of democracy.

In 21st century the feminist literature reached a paradigmatic stage. The global issues pertaining to women have been pursued from political, social, cultural, economic, developmental, ecological and psychological perspectives. But issues pertaining to women with disabilities have not been approached and to think even of paradigms in the context of disabled women is a very distant dream. It would be clichéd to state that women form the 'marginal component' of society. What is ironical in case of this group virtually that even the number of disabled women is not known. (Meenu, 2003)

Policies and Programmes: Himachal in Focus

John Rawals is well known for his theory of justice and still considered as the one of the most authoritative theorists on justice. But Rawals ignored gender in his theory of justice. For a feminist critic of Rawals theory of justice, S.M. Okin has argued that under the Rawalsian paradigm, injustice against women within the household is invisible. Justice if not viewed within the family can only result in strengthening patriarchal norms (Okin, 1989). We have noted that the specificity of disabled women status has been linked to the general group of disable, thus meeting the legitimacy of their claims to the experiences of different disabilities, for instance, those with hearing problems have commonality of issue, which are not gendered. We realized that within this setting, the placing of women within the general understanding of disability sector, whether visual, locomotors or any other is fragmented, as far as they were seen with gendered lenses. The disability alone categorization was therefore insufficient to understand their problems. This is proved by the fact that disabled women are nearly invisible element, not only in the general disability movement but more so in the women's movement. Through our experiences of working with the disability sector, we have realized that women within the disability movement, at least in the initial phase, are included because it is politically correct to include women then for any other reason.

While as women they face similar problem, as disabled women they experience problems different from the non-disabled. Therefore, their problems need to be addressed by both the feminist and disability movement. Despite this, within the women movement at large they remained rightly invisible. In the context of women with disabilities, the volume therefore attempts to provide a comparative, relational based conception of feminism, which has been excluded from the general majority of a global feminist literature and movement. We believe these women are overlooked, this regarded and neglected as a group within majority of feminists' strategies. The Constitution of India ensures quality, freedom, justice and dignity of all individuals and implicitly mandates an inclusive society for all including persons with disabilities. The framers of the constitution were well aware of the fact that in the process of providing true equality some benefits would have to be given to certain sections of the society. Articles 14, 15 and 16 of the Constitution of India clearly recognize this concept and Article 41 of the Constitution of India states that the State shall, within the limits of its economic capacity and development concomitant to these provisions, in 1995 Parliament has passed an act called People With Disability Act (PWD Act, 1995) for the all round protection and promotion of disabled community rights "THE PERSONS WITH DISABILITIES" Act, 1995 was brought into force from the 1st of January, 1996.

According to this Act, 3 per cent reservation has to be provided to disabled community in all government employment. Today after 15 years of the compliance of the Act, it has not been implemented in its true proportion in any department either with the central or state governments. So is the state of many other developmental welfare schemes targeted for the betterment of the disabled people. The national policy on disability, 2006 mandated each state to have its own State Disability Policy (SDP) though it was promised in 2008 that the state will have its own SDP, yet it has taken a long time for the hilly State to have its own SDP. Himachal Pradesh has come out with its first SDP for persons with disability, the policy is approved by state cabinet and was notified on March 10, 2011. Himachal has become the sixth state after Goa, Karnataka, Tamil Nadu, Orissa and Chhattisgarh to have its own State Disability Policy. The policy sums up all dimensions based upon a social human right model, focusing on capabilities and inclusion of PWDs calling for mitigating the environmental and attitudinal barriers along with providing for educational employment opportunities with an aim to mainstream PWDs. The policy visions an involvement of actors outside the core framework including NGOs and PRIs in implementation and intervention. The policy also stress on the access of education to disables in mainstream schools, and home based education depending upon the level of disability. (*TOI*, 17 March 2011, p. 6). In the state 11,871 disable children and 2,284 are special children who are not in the position to go to schools, to educate them quality education plan '*adhar*' has been implemented to give them education involving 550 NGOs. The teachers will be specially trained and equipped to teach them. (*Amar Ujjala*, 2011) Sarv Shiksha Abhiyan (SSA) had identified 22044 Children With Special Needs (CWSN), which is 2.34 per cent of the total school going children at elementary level.

At present, 19643 CWSN have been integrated in formal schools and for 2397 out of school CWSN, different strategies have been adopted to bring them in education system. (*TOI*, 2011)

The social model of disability allows the possibility that disability or social oppression may or may not exist in any particular context, or that may exist differently across cultures and over time. In separating the individual body/mind from social responses to the body/mind, it becomes possible to unlock the different dimensions of disability that exist in different cultures and communities (Emma Stone, 2001). Disable people are marginalized but women within disability are worse. Women are doubly discriminated one as a disabled and another as a women. The state of overall women in our country is pathetic and women with disability are subjected to variety of societal and governmental apathies. There are several other domains of women where neglect has been perpetuated by all corners against them both by the society as well as by the state. But the status of women with disabilities are extremely pathetic and need urgent attention by all concerned. At all India level, the states of women with disabilities are not at par with able women. It is also pertinent to mention here that without bringing women with disabilities into the mainstreaming process of development, we could not ensure the real concept of sustainable development. With this angle of development there is an urgent need to look into women with disabilities with separate identity within disability. Inclusion of this component is required to accommodate not only into the planning process but in its implementation too. Given the enormity of this issue the focus of 2011 census in on gender sensitization and disability data. The needs of the disables were put on low priority because people with disability are invisible only 2 out of 10 persons are counted in census 2001, this is indicative of the fact that majority of people with disability are still hidden. To get the person with disability counted question no. 9 of census of India 2011is on disability where 8 types of disability has been mentioned. The special training was given to the enumerators to elicit the answer for this question. In Himachal Pradesh the Persons with disability (PWDs) constitutes 2 per cent (1,55,950 persons) of the total population including all categories of persons with impairment irrespective of degree of impairment as compared to national no of 2.19 crore which constitutes 2.13 per cent of total population of India. It is very evident from the available data that number of disables is more in rural area (75 per cent) as compared to urban area and about 49 per cent PWDs are literate rest are illiterate.

The National and State policies and programmes for disables recognize that persons with disability are valuable human resource for the country. The majority of persons with disability can lead better quality of life if environment is created to provide them equal opportunities, protection of their rights and full participation in society. It is worth mentioning here that Himachal Pradesh has been ranked to be the Jt. First among the states in the country in implementation of the provisions of the Persons With Disabilities Act, 1995 (Equal Opportunities, Protection of Rights, and Full participation).

The government of Himachal Pradesh has also implemented National Trust for welfare of people of persons with Autism, cerebral Palsy, Mental Retardation and Multiple Disability Act, 1999. This Act has provisions for providing legal guardianship to people suffering from Autism, cerebral Palsy, Mental Retardation and Multiple Disability and for creation of an enabling environment to make them more independent. The National Trust Act, 1999 is being implemented in the state and Local Level Committees have been constituted in all 12 districts of the State and legal guardians for the persons with these disabilities are being appointed. The solemn efforts of the State for mainstreaming of PWDs envisage:

- Prevention of Disabilities.
- Rehabilitation of persons with Disabilities.
- Enabling Environment for the Persons with Disabilities.

As per provisions of Persons with Disability Act, 1995, 3 per cent reservation is provided in government jobs in class A to D posts. The reservation is further divided amongst visually, hearing and orthopaedically impaired person 15 each. From the year 2007 to 2011 jobs given to visually impaired is 421 persons, 293 to hearing impaired and 550 for orthopaedically impaired persons. In the span of four years total of 1264 jobs were given in the public sector. The age-wise survey of PWDs in the state shows that maximum number of impairment is orthopedic and number of disabled person in each category of impairments increases with increase in age. The potential causes of orthopedic impairment include genetic abnormality, diseases, injury, birth trauma, amputation, burns or other causes. The polio virus is major cause of orthopedic disability and threat to humanity worldwide. According to business magnate turned philanthropist Bill Gates explained that India can achieve zero transmission of polio in next two years. India which is considered as hotbed of polio virus had reduced the cases substantially from 741 in 2009 to 42 in 2010 which shows 94 per cent decline in polio cases. The government of Himachal Pradesh has implemented various schemes for the welfare of persons with disability where government and various NGOs are hand in hand. The disable persons having disability of 40% or above and whose annual income does not exceed Rs. 6,000 individually and Rs. 11,000 (along with family), are provided Disability Relief Allowance (DRA) @ Rs. 330 per month. At present 28,867 number of disabled persons are getting DRA in the State. Many institutions and NGOs are engaged in working in disability. They are encouraged and facilitated to play effective role to complement the efforts of government. The NGOs have significant advisory role in planning, policy formulation, implementation and information sharing on best practices.

The earlier emphasis on medical rehabilitation has now been replaced by an emphasis on social rehabilitation. There has been an increasing recognition of abilities of persons with disabilities and emphasis on mainstreaming them in the society based on their capabilities. Recent postmodern Sociology has generated a tendency to pit fluid, contextual notions of individual lived experiences against fixed and rigid notions of social structure. The development of disabled people's movement individual and collective efforts of abled and disabled people can bring about real change in societies and in individual people's lives.

Concluding Remarks

For the better future of mankind, it is both economically unsound and morally unacceptable to ignore the potential contribution that disable women can make in the wider society in and outside their homes. They cannot be excluded from equal participation in mainstream society. It must be recognized that all people with or without disability are unique. At the same time it is also true that the presence of disability, especially severe life impacting disabilities that required the assistance of others in order to navigate the daily tasks of living, create a level of vulnerability, not experienced by people without disabilities. The people with disabilities, particularly women are collectively defined as a social monolith. In quantum Physics, 'super symmetry' is prerequisite for perfect condition but that is far from reality. But we cannot access this reality if mind is functioning in the same way as it now. It has to function from a different level. And what is that level, where there is no knowledge and no ignorance. (*TOI*, 2011). The contractarian logic of justice, as enunciated in Rawls, does not adequately address the question of inequality producing persistent injustices in an otherwise just society and polity. Probably overall stress on the distribution on primarily goods fails to build capabilities in a manner as to reduce injustices. The capability approach as developed by Amartya Sen primarily emphasizes the expansion of opportunities then recommending particular framework of policy. "The capability approach," writes Amartya Sen, "focuses on human life, and not just on some detached objects of inconvenience, such as incomes or commodities that a person may possess... The focus of the capability approach is thus not just on what a person actually ends up doing, but also she is in fact able to do...". (Amartya Sen, 2009, pp. 233-234)

As we enter the third millennium, concern about the social and political dimensions of disablement has intensified considerably. The exclusion of disabled people from the mainstream of economic and social life has been the subject of mounting political protest and mobilization. It has become major issue for policy makers and politicians in developed and developing countries alike and growing number have introduced some form of legislative framework in which to combat discrimination on the grounds of impairment or disability. A sociological approach suggests that the common meanings associated with impairment and disability emerged out of specific social and cultural context. Disability does not have a universal character. During the 1970s and 1980s, disabled activists and their organizations voiced increasing criticism of the individual, disability model of disabling, disabled people argued that it is society which disables people with impairments, and therefore any meaningful solution must be directed to develop a social model for change rather than individual adjustment and rehabilitation.

The shift from the medical and charity models to the social model of disability will be an undeniable progress. However there is the danger of taxing vegetate in rhetoric and truism about societal discrimination and marginalization, while some sociological realities are not properly understood or keenly taken into account. It is important to consider the material and mental barriers such as poverty, hardship and internalized negative attitudes from within because if we have to go further in the social model and achieve sustainable changes, the family environment is unavoidable. The discourse on conceptualizing disability shows that the status of women with disabilities can never be truly understood until we understand the complexity, that is, disability. It is not possible to deny how important the ideological, economic and social structures of the society are when defining the term in effect demarcating the position of those who are so defined. The dilemma of whether the problem lies within the individual or the environment will perhaps be clarified only when research is conducted and the experiences of persons with disabilities are analyzed.

The exclusion of disabled women in the mainstream of society has led to the society being the poorer in terms of skills and experiences. Many efforts are now being made by the government and disabled persons themselves to improve the situation. However it is imperative that the government takes forward the policy governing the employment, rehabilitation etc. (Asha, 2003) There is no country in the world where disabled people's rights are not violated. The discrimination, oppression, violence and abuse faced by disabled people does not respect national boundaries, national wealth or national poverty. The right based strategies for development and social change are what is needed and development of disabled people's movement and individual and collective efforts of abled and disabled people can bring real attitudinal, institutional and radical change in the society. The problem of disability is all about commonality – not a commonality of embodied experiences but commonality of purpose, in the struggle for a more inclusive society. The disables should fully participate in identifying their own needs, goals, programme plans and the contexts in which strategies, policies and programmes will be carried out.

It has been concluded from the study undertaken that Himachal Pradesh is doing better than any other state of the country as far as governmental efforts are concerned. It has not only implemented these welfare measures for the capacity building but has also created conducive environment for their better human development index. But the status of women with disability, which is the focal agenda of discussion of this paper, is far better than its counterparts in rest of the parts of the country but for the realization of an ideal situation women should be included as special group within the disabled community.

REFERENCES

1. *Amar Ujjala*, Shimla, March 7, 2011, p. 1.
2. Annual Report on Disability (2009-10), Department of Social Justice and Empowerment, Govt. of Himachal Pradesh.
3. Asha Hans and Annie Patri (2003), Women, Disability and Identity, Sage Publications, New Delhi.
4. Casteel, C., Martin, *et al* (2008), National Study of physical and sexual assault among women with disabilities. Inj Prev. 14(2), 87-90.
5. Cathy McPherson (1991), 'Violence as it affects Disabled Women' in *Women and Disability*, Boylan Esther (ed.) Zed Books Ltd. London.
6. Coleridge, P. (1993), *Disability, Liberation and Development,* Oxfame Publishing, Oxford.
7. Emma, Stone (2001), *A Complicated Struggle: Disability, Survival and Social Change in the Majority World* in Mark Priestley (ed.) University Press, Cambridge.
8. Mark Priestly (ed.) (2001), Disability and The Life Course, University Press, Cambridge.
9. Meenu Bhambani (2003), Societal Responses to Women with Disabilities in India in Asha Hans, *op cit.*, No. 11.
10. National Policy for Persons with Disability (2006), Ministry of Social Justice and Empowerment, *GOI*, New Delhi.

11. Okin, S.M.(1989), *Justice, Gender and the Family*, New York,
12. Olsvile, V.M. (2006), Vulnerable, exposed and invisible: a study of violence and abuse against women with physical disabilities, *Scand. J. Disabil. Res.* 8(2), 85-96.
13. Polly Vizard (2006), Poverty and Human Rights, Oxford University Press, New Delhi,
14. Sen, Amartya (2009), *The Idea of Justice*, Penguin, London, pp. 233-34.
15. *Times of India*, Chandigarh, March 17, 2011, p. 6.
16. United Nations Children's Fund, 1999.
17. UPIAS/Disability Aliance (1976), Fundamental Principles of Disability, UPIAS, Disability Aliance, London.

14

Disability and Gender: Indian Context

Sudhir Kumar Singh

Disability is part and parcel of every society. Its roots could be traced back to evolution of human race. Since the inception of the human race there has been a gap of resources between rich and the poor. At the out set of 21st century it has been further aggravated with the free flow of the tenets of globalization. But these prevailing imbalances into their resources could not only reflect with the status of the people with disability but it has doubly making an impact on the community. Disability is a point of discrimination in all societies either it is developed or developing countries. It is particularly a matter of social stigma which prevails since centuries. In developing countries too they are confronting with gamut of discrimination embedded with social stigmas. According to International Groups of Disabled Rights "In our view, it is society which disables.... Disability is something imposed on top of our impairments, by the way we are unnecessarily isolated and excluded from full participation in society. Disabled people are therefore an oppressed group in society."[1]

In developing countries the situation of common development has remained pathetic due to variety if reasons. Majority of developing countries have emerged independent after the Second World War. Many among them have adopted democracy as the way of governance. Democracy insists on the common development with special component of the development to the marginalized. In a broader term it is called inclusive growth. Simply it means to bring all segments of the society together into the developmental process. By all cannons of social justice, the disability includes as one of the worst group within marginalized groups. The component of human rights has emerged as one of the most publicized agenda of the international system with the end of the cold war. It has further expanded in post-9/11 international scenario. Human rights and democracy however are dependent on each other. In other words human rights could not be realized in the absence of democratic framework. Because with the component of social and economic rights the beauty of democracy is to provide civil and political rights to the people on the basis of equality. But even in democracies, which are morally compelled to implement the egalitarian agenda of human rights, it is observed that it has kept mum on the compliance of these cardinal principles of democracy. Today right from the Egypt to Libya, the wave of democratization is extremely intense. But the United States which consider itself as one of the important harbingers of the global democracy regime could not pursued this agenda into its vessel clients State like Saudi Arabia due to maximize its vested agenda. India is considered as one of the largest democracies of the world but in the case of Burma it has not been able to promote democratic values despite severe torture to democratic activists by military junta it is engaging the Junta to maximize its national interest to contain the influence of its arch rival China there. But despite these isolated infringements these countries have expressed their desire to support democratic values across the globe. Post-cold war and post-9/11 international system has further aggravated this wave of democratization and human rights. Disability is one of the most vital human concern and 1993 Vienna Convention of international human rights have first time adopted disability as one of the most crucial component and more than 150 countries of the contemporary world are signatories of this declaration. Again under the aegis of the U.N. majority of world governments have signed the declarations which ensure the compliance of all rights to disables in 2007. Globally it has been established as one of the most deprived sector of the humanity therefore beside many international laws, many municipal laws have also been enacted for the promotion and protection of the rights of the disable community.

Disable people as part of the society deserve equal rights like able people. They are not asking for any charity but just asking for equal rights to realize their eternal urge of equality which has remained as one of the most important cardinal principle of democratic rights from the French Revolution of 1789. The United States has been claiming since a long time that it is the sole harbinger of the international regime of human rights. But even with the end of cold war, when communism has been evaporated from the universe, the United States despite their rhetoric of human rights have extended all round support to many authoritarian regimes for the sake of their national interests. Despite these prevailing realities, it is a fact that with the process of globalization human rights have become one of the most important components of international system. Even authoritarian regimes have become compelled to pay lip services to the cause.

For democracy as I have stated earlier it is the life blood to provide all kinds of amenities to the common people with exclusive stress on destitute. Kautilaya, the great Indian Philosopher has insisted in his famous book *Arthsastra* that a king must nurture their subject as a new born baby is nurtured by his/her mother. One could trace the origins of democracy and human rights from his writing. He was the prime minister of the greatest Indian empire called Mauryan Empire. We are aware about the fact that monarchy was not accountable for the people because merely it was of the opinion that it derives its legitimacy of rule from the almighty god therefore it is only accountable for god. In democracy, people are the custodian therefore the elected ruler must be accountable for the people and people are most benefited element by all theoretical frameworks. But in reality prevalence of chronic poverty across the globe particularly in less developed and developing countries exclusively in those countries which have adopted democracy as a mode of governance is a blatant denial of the fundamental rights of the common people.

In many developing countries it is matter of governance but in majority of them lack of resources and rampant corruption is denying the basic tenets of democracy to the common people.

It almost fits into the Indian context. India is a developing country and recently World Bank has announced that within next two years, India will be surpassing China is GDP growth.[2] Despite being a newly emerged country, India has done tremendous progress in all round development. Today after six decade of our independence, one of the biggest concerns remains and that is inclusion of the marginalized into the mainstreaming process of development. It is one of the most crucial factors, which sustains a kind of unrest in our society. Poverty is a great denial of democracy and human rights. It is true that since last few decades we have been able to upgrade the life standard of 300 million people. But according to the Planning Commission still around 35 per cent people lives below the poverty line. According to the 2011 census, India has 121 crore population and still existing gender gap vindicates the point that gender has been discriminated despite growing literacy and prosperity. Currently 11th Five Year Plan (2007-12) is in operation. According to the Approach Paper of the 11th Plan "The 11th Plan provides an opportunity to restructure policies to achieve a new vision of growth that would be much more broad based and inclusive, bringing about a faster reduction in poverty and helping bridge the divides that are currently the focus of so much attention. The first steps in this direction were initiated in the middle of the Tenth Plan based on the National Common Minimum Programme adopted by the government. These steps must be further strengthened and consolidated into a strategy for the 11th Plan."[3]

The Approach Paper of the 11th Plan stressed on gender development. According to the paper, "The gender divide is another dimension of the problem which needs urgent attention. Gender bias is deeply ingrained in our society and is reflected in indicators like sex ratios, literacy levels of boys and girls, Maternal Mortality Rates (MMR), etc. however, even these data do not fully reflect the discrimination against women. The 11th Plan strategy for gender balancing must take care of the special needs of women such as clean cooking fuels, care for pregnant and nursing women etc. Gender balancing would require appropriate provisions in government policies/schemes across Ministries/Departments and sectors."[4]

We are aware about the census data 2011. It reveals that gender ratio is decreasing despite positive indications from other realm of human development. If the status of common women has not been improved then what about women with disability. They are forced to face barrage of hostilities despite that the fact that India is growing as an economic power at the global stage. Poverty is rampant and empirical experience reveals that poverty hamper's the aspiration of the people with disability in general and women with disability in particular.

Nobel Laureate Prof. Amartya Sen has advanced international thinking about global poverty as a human rights issue. Sen's work in ethics and economics has emerged as a key influence on international decades about global poverty and human rights, and has depended and expanded theoretical thinking about this issue in important and innovative ways. Global poverty has moved rapidly up to the international human rights agenda in recent years. Virtually all governments have recognized the protection and promotion of human rights aimed at survival and human development including the human rights to life, the human rights to a standard of living adequate for health and well being and the human right to education-as ethical, legal, political and economic imperatives for the 21st century. Global poverty causes these internationally recognized human rights to be violated and denied and has been described by Mary Robinson, the former United Nations high commissioner for human Rights, as the worst human rights problem the world faces today.[5] There are inherent relationship between disability and poverty. Disable community requires better medical attention and poverty prevents them to avail this urgent need. It has resulted into the variety of hazards for the people of disability, the most important component within marginalized groups. According to the international agencies, the number of disable people in India is 8-10 per cent but government of India insists that they are less than 3 per cent only. Here lies the seed of discrimination of people with disability. Disable people constitute sizable portion of our population but due to governmental apathy their welfare schemes are inadequate, which kept them excluded despite all round claim of the government about their development.

India could not be strong without accommodating disable population into the mainstreaming process of development into the 21st century. Disable community remains one of the most discriminated in Indian context because of discrimination. India is a country where even at the out set of the 21st century societal support or opposition matters for the formation and implementation of any legislation of any nature. Disable community is confronting with the societal stigma. Because society still plays extremely important role in our system therefore disable people's all round development has been jeopardized.

Noted disable rights activist, Anita Ghai has cited one worst experience of a disable person and according to her "Destiny, fate, god, past sins ... Call it whatever you will ... it is not justified ... it would have been better if I had been allowed one day instead of dying everyday". [Lakhmi][6]

Activist and scholars have acknowledged the expanding of borders of feminist research to include women with class, ethnic, national and other diversities. The widening sphere means that awareness about women problems in many sectors including the home, the workplace and other domains are slowly and steadily unveiled before us. In spite of the increasing range of issues that are being recognized as important, we note that a space for disabled women has yet to be found in serious feminist research. We discovered that as social group disabled women have hardly found a place in any existing theory. This reduced us to conclude that we need a space demarcated for women with disabilities in present day researches.

John Rawals is well known for his theory of justice and still considered as the one of the most authoritative theorist on justice. But Rawal's ignored gender in his theory of justice. For a feminist critic of Rawal's theory of justice, S.M. Okin has argued that under the Rawlinson paradigm, injustice against women within the house hold is invisible. Justice if not viewed within the family can only result in strengthening patriarchal norms.[7] We noted that the specificity of disabled women status has been linked to the general group of disable, thus meeting the legitimacy of their claims to the experiences of different disabilities, for instance, those with hearing problems have commonality of issue, which are not gendered. We realized that within this setting, the placing of women within the general understanding of disability sector, whether visual, locomotors or any other is fragmented, as far as they were seen with gendered lenses. The disability alone categorization was therefore insufficient to understand their problems. This is proved by the fact that disabled women are nearly invisible element, not only in the general disability movement but more so in the women's movement. Through our experiences of working with the disability sector, we have realized that women within the disability movement, at least in the initial phase, are included because of some vested interests.

While as women they face similar problem, as disabled women they experience problems different from the non-disabled. Therefore, their problems need to be addressed by both the feminist and disability movement. Despite this, we noticed that within the women movement at large they remained rightly invisible. In the context of women with disabilities, the contemporary debate therefore attempts to provide a comparative, relational based conception of feminism, which has been excluded from the general majority of a global feminist literature and movement. We believe these women are overlooked, this regarded and neglected as a group within majority of feminists strategies.

In 1995, Parliament has passed an act called People With Disability Act (PWD Act, 1995) for the all round protection and promotion of disable community rights. According to this Act, 3 per cent reservation has to be provided to disable community in all government employment but till date the true essence of its implementation is missing. So is the state of many other developmental welfare schemes targeted for the betterment of the disabled people.

Disable people are marginalized but women within disability are worse because they are discriminated disabled and another women. The state of overall women in our country is pathetic and women with disability are subjected to variety of societal and governmental apathy's. There are several other domains of women where neglect has been perpetuated by all corners against them both by the society as well as by the state. But the status of women with disabilities is extremely pathetic and need urgent attention by all concerned. At all India level, the status of women with disabilities is not at par with able women. It is also pertinent to mention here that without bringing women with disabilities into the mainstreaming process of development, we could not ensure the real concept of sustainable development. With this angle of development there is an urgent need to look into women with disabilities with separate identity within disability. Inclusion of this component is required to accommodate not into the planning process but in its implementation too. For this purpose a broad based awareness is badly required. Given the enormity of this issue this paper will try to cover the status of disable women in India.

Disability is a feminist issue, but is largely ignored in citizenship debates. Disability is gendered, affecting men and women differently. A process of exclusion diminishes the well-being of both those affected and those, who consciously or unconsciously, participate in such a process. Women with disabilities/disabled women, largely inhabiting these margins, may experience the illusion of inclusion. The public imagination conceives of most people with disabilities, especially women, as passive citizens. They represent a source of increasing demand for services in an environment of ever-diminishing state and public finances. Dominant ideologies within the disability arena are changing from welfare to rights, yet people with disabilities still do not appear as active members of the community. Forced to claim 'special rights', their status as citizens with existing rights (albeit unacknowledged/inaccessible) is negated. Their rights however have emerged as an important concern for the state as well as the civil-society. But in a country like India, it is extremely turbulent that their genuine citizenry rights have been in fringed. First it will be established than one could process their exclusive rights. Although they have emerged a critical arena of international human rights regime but it has not been translated into action despite many legislation and civil-society efforts. One could not separate the status of women with disability with the status of common women in Indian society.

People who experience disability find themselves propelled from the 'normal' range of taken-for-granted 'rights', into the realm of passivity and lack of agency. Downward social mobility and social status often converge with acquired disability status.[8] Since Athenian times, men with disabilities, along with women, slaves and so on, have been excluded by law from citizenship status, physically prevented from taking any active role in democratic societies or indirectly constrained by discriminatory and oppressive institutions and ideologies. At one extreme they have been viewed as sub-human – 'freaks' – and, like some indigenous people, the objects of extermination policies, justified through 'scientific' discourses. Recently a more benevolent and enlightened approach has seen the construction of people with disabilities as fully human and 'capable' of some assimilation into mainstream society. Efforts have been made in India both by the state and the civil-society to mainstreaming gender disability into the developmental as well into the planning process. But fact of the matter is that disability as a component has yet to include into the mainstreaming process despite gamut of assurances. First it needs to be incorporated than the women with disability will be better justified.

Now the question arises that how we will be bringing women with disabilities into the mainstreaming process. There may be variety of measures for the achievement of this goal but the most practical is there empowerment. The researches in this arena carried out by many agencies have insisted that majority of disable people are able to work without any aid and appliances. If we will provide them employment than they will not only able to earn their bread and expanses for medical requirements but could promote the overall movement of disability too. This aspect is extremely important for the women with disabilities. Their employment will give them self-confidence to their personality and they will act with better confidence to cope all challenges in their life. There are multiple perspectives on empowerment and the particular meanings given to the construct, according to persons, settings, goals, and other variables. Research on empowerment has largely focused on groups that are typically considered disadvantaged, disempowered or ostensibly powerless[9] Luke, Rappaport, and Seidman[10] suggested that empowerment is more than a mere process, solution, or exemplar as is, for instance, prevention. Instead, they posit that empowerment is the process to which the primary energies of psychologists, counselors, social workers, and others should be directed and through which most of the goals for social and individual change will be most appropriately accomplished. Zimmerman and Warschausky, in their rehabilitation research, asserted further that a focus on individual or person-centered notions of empowerment precludes us from seeing the implications for community or social change. Empowerment, they argue, should not be treated simply as some personality variable that would neglect the construct's social relationship. For instance, among service providers to mentally disabled clients, empowerment has become a program principle[11] that underlies group self-help designs, mechanisms and consequences. Nobel Laureate, Amartya Sen has also argued that incorporation of gender into the mainstreaming of development is the key to the success of the initiative of human development for any society. The government of India has already started the process but it has yet to take off properly and component of disability is absent from this debate. It is vindicated only with one fact that government of India counts disable community as merely 2.3 per cent of total population despite the fact that UN agencies are often mentioning that it is not less than 10 per cent. Here lies the crux of the problem because when government will not accept their real number it means that the planning process will allocate resources in a different manner. Needless to say that it has marred the prospects of the actual empowerment of the disable community, which remains as a severe issue of concern for our desired goal of sustainable development. When in totality disable community has not been given its due share than asking for separate arrangements for the women with disabilities seems to a castles in the air.

However given the actual situation at the grass root level in India, we have to formulate our strategies to cope with the situation under which women with disability get benefited. First of all poverty is important in the context. Planning Commission has accepted that around 35 per cent people are below poverty line and numbers of welfare measures have been carried out to bring them from this deprived situation. But here again governmental apathy remains matter for grave concern for all concerned. For example, the government has given exclusive attention for the plight of the SC/ST community through a number of corrective measures. But at the same time, it has not been much concerned for the same level of efforts for the welfare of disable community. One could trace this imbalance within the governmental policies regarding resource allocation for the welfare of the disable community. The fact is the government data, itself insisted that there is strong link between disability and social marginalization. The NSSO data 1991 suggests that 40 per cent of the disable poor belong to the SC/ST community. Thus, if empowerment schemes of the SC/ST do not have a disability component, a large section of the community will be deliberately doomed to marginalization.

In Indian context, where poverty is rampant and traverse all artificial barriers, better employment opportunities could improve their situation in a massive manner probably by the enactment of 1995 People With Disability by the parliament, which provide 3 per cent reservation in all governmental services to the people with disabilities. But the majority of people with disabilities particularly women with disabilities didn't have adequate educational as well technological qualification therefore they are not eligible for these positions. Majority of women with disabilities are from unorganized sector and particularly from the enormously vast rural sector. The work activity status of disabled persons depicts that about 46 per cent of disabled populations both in rural and urban areas were without work. Only 1.8 and 7.3 per cent disable persons in rural and urban areas respectively were regular employees in 2002. Even the nature was only in low profile jobs with bare minimum income. Provide employment opportunities for disable persons is the top priority to make them self-reliant. Unfortunately, very few employment opportunities are provided to the disable persons due to social, cultural and work potential bias against them. It is more suited for the denial of job opportunities for the women with disabilities. The National Centre for Promotion of Employment for Disabled Persons (NCPEDP) in collaboration with the National Association for Blind, Delhi, conducted a survey for disabled persons since the enactment of PWD Act, 1995.[12] The survey was conducted in 119 NGOs. major findings of the surveys are as follows:

- Only 12.89 per cent disabled people were among the professional staff members of these organizations. Disabled women again formed a dismal 4.47 per cent of the group. The administrative structure of the respondent organizations seems to be dominated by non-disabled males.
- About 50 per cent of the disabled people placed by the respondent organization in the last two years were self-employed. Only 1/4 of the beneficiaries were disable women.
- According to the data, about 90 per cent of the people were earning less than 2,000 per month. In fact, 47.50 per cent of them earn below Rs. 1,000 per month.
- Though 1,628 private sector companies were approached in the last two years for placement by the respondent organization, only 1,557 disabled people found jobs in this sector. While 804 public sector companies were approached, only 220 disabled people get jobs in this sector for the last two years.
- Only 33.61 per cent of the respondents organizations register their beneficiaries with employment exchanges. Only 212 disabled people were placed through this channel out of the total job placement of 4,812 disabled persons.
- While 5,618 disabled people received vocational training in the last one year, only 4,812 people were placed in the last two years.
- Only a handful of organizations provide training in industry related skills to disabled people. Majority of the NGOs provide training in skills like art and crafts, making stationery item's etc, which limit their options to self-employment.

Concluding Remarks

India is sustaining a high pace of growth since last many years despite odd global scenario. In the contemporary world, beside China there is hardly any country which could equate Indian pace of all round development. But the fact remains that women remains at the receiving end by any parameter of human development index than man and even 2011 census data proves this argument. Women need to be included into the mainstreaming process of development than only the real concept of sustainable development could be achieved. As far as women with disability is concerned there problem is twin first as a women and second as a disable. For the proper mitigation of the challenges we need to develop the capacity level of the women with disability. As NSSO data reveals they are able to work and we know that they need better medicinal as well as societal attention for the betterment of their life therefore we need to ensure their economic empowerment. Merely governmental sector is unable to provide this opportunity to one of the most hapless segment of our society. It needs all concerned efforts and we must do this. Private sector will be a great help. We need to harness the concept of corporate social responsibility because due to the growing clout of the process of globalization, market forces are strengthening and they need to allocate adequate resources for this unfortunate section of our society. Only all concerned sincere efforts could ensure all round well being of the women with disability. Being a democratic society we need to implement all legislation for the promotion and protection of the cause. Since we believe in the concept of welfare state therefore it is the duty of the society to provide basic societal support to women with disability. Our traditional values propelled us to extend all possible support to women but women with disability need more support from the society than the government because government neither could nor be successful till we will not provide positive support to women with disability. At the outset of the 21st century it is an open secret that women with disability in particular live not at par with common citizens of our country. They are asking for parity not for charity and we need to realize this fact in a candid manner. Societal awareness could be pivotal for the compliance of this egalitarian goal. The consciousness is increasing in this field but more needs to be done to provide tenets of human rights to women with disability.

REFERENCES

1. UPIAS/Disability Aliance, Fundamental Principles of Disability, UPIAS, Disability Aliance, 1976, London.
2. *Times of India*, New Delhi, January 2011.
3. Towards Faster and More Inclusive Growth; An Approach to the 11th Five Year Plan, Planning Commission, Government of India, New Delhi, 2006, p.1.
4. Ibid., p. 64.
5. Robinson, Mary (2004) Health, Human Rights and Development, OECD Forum. Available at http://www.oecd.org/dataoecd/7/27/31787614.pdf.
6. Marginalization and Disability, Experiences from the Third World, Anita Ghai in Disability and Life Course; Global Perspectives (eds) Mark Priestley, Cambridge University Press, Cambridge, 2001.
7. Okin, S.M. (1989) Justice, Gender and the Family, New York, Basic Books.
8. Jenkins, R. (1991) 'Disability and social stratification', *British Journal of Sociology*, Vol. 42, No. 4: 557-80.
9. Thompson, S.C., Spacapan, S. (1991) Perceptions of control in vulnerable populations. J. Soc. Iss. 47(4), 1–21.
10. Luke, D.A., Rappaport, J., Seidman, E. (2002) Setting Phenotypes in a Mutual Help Organization: Expanding Behavior Setting Theory, pp. 217–238.
11. Cohen, M.B. (1989) Social work practice with homeless mentally ill people: engaging the client. *Social Work*, 34(6), 505–509.
12. Role of NGOs vis-a-vis The Employment Scenario in India with reference to people with Disabilities, NCPEDP and The National Association for the Blind, Delhi Research Study.

Bibliography

Ablon, J. (1984). *Little people in America: The social dimensions of Dwarfism.* New York: Praeger Publishers.

Adams, R. (2001). *Sideshow U.S.A.: Freaks and the American cultural imagination.* Chicago: University of Chicago Press.

Ahern, L., and Rosenthal, E., with Bauer, E., Calik, N., Kanter, A., Layikel, Okain, R., & Sundram, C. (2005). *Behind closed doors: Human rights abuses in the psychiatric facilities, orphanages and rehabilitation centers of Turkey.* Washington, DC: Mental Disability Rights International.

Albrecht, G. L. (1992). *The disability business: Rehabilitation in America* [Sage Library of Social Research Vol. 190]. Newbury Park: Sage Publications.

Albrecht, G. L., Seelman, K. D., and Bury, M. (Eds.). (2001). *Handbook of disability studies.* Thousand Oaks, CA: Sage Publications.

Allard, M. A., Howard, A. M., Vorderer, L. E., and Wells, A. I. (1999). *Ahead of his time: Selected speeches of Gunnar Dybwad.* Washington, DC: American Association on Mental Retardation.

Barnartt, S., and Scotch, R. (2001). *Disability protests: Contentious politics 1970-1999.* Washington, DC: Gallaudet University Press.

Barnes, C., and Mercer, G. (2003). *Disability* [Key Concepts]. Cambridge, United Kingdom: Polity Press.

Barnes, C., Oliver, M., and Barton, L. (Eds.). (2002). *Disability Studies today.* Cambridge, United Kingdom: Polity Press.

Baynton, D. C. (1996). *Forbidden signs: American culture and the campaign against sign language.* Chicago: University Of Chicago Press.

Becker, G. (1978). *The mad genius controversy: A study in the sociology of deviance* [Sociological Observations]. Beverly Hills, CA: Sage Publications.

Behuniak, S. M., and Svenson, A. G. (2003). *Physician-assisted suicide: The anatomy of a constitutional law issue.* Lanham, MD: Rowman & Littlefield Publishers, Inc.

Ben-Moshe, L., Cory, R. C., Feldbaum, M., and Sagendorf, K. (Eds.). (2005). *Building pedagogical curb cuts: Incorporating disability in the university classroom and curriculum.* Syracuse, NY: The Graduate School, Syracuse University.

Berube, M. (1996). *Life as we know it: A father, a family, and an exceptional child.* New York: Random House.

Biklen, D., with Attfield, R., Bissonnette, L., Blackman, L., Burke, J., & Frugone, A. (2005). *Autism and the myth of the person alone* (Qualitative Studies in Psychology). New York: NYU Press.

Blanck, P., Hill, E., Siegal, C. D., and Waterstone, M. (2004). *Disability civil rights law and policy* [Hornbook Series]. St. Paul: Thomson West.

Bogdan, R. (1988). *Freak show: Presenting human oddities for amusement and profit.* Chicago: University of Chicago Press.

Bogdan, R., and Taylor, S. J. (1994). *The social meaning of mental retardation: Two life stories* [Special Education Series]. New York: Teachers College Press.

Branson, J., and Miller, D. (2002). *Damned for their difference: The cultural construction of Deaf people as disabled: A sociological history.* Washington, DC: Gallaudet University Press.

Braginsky, D. D., and Braginsky, B. M. (1971). *Hansels and Gretels: Studies of children in institutions for the mentally retarded.* New York: Holt, Rinehart and Winston, Inc.

Breslin, M. L., and Yee, S. (Eds.). (2002). *Disability rights law and policy: International and national perspectives.* Ardsley, NY: Transnational Publishers.

Brown, S. E. (2000). *A celebration of diversity: An annotated bibliography about disability culture.* Las Cruces, NM: Institute on Disability Culture.

Campbell, J., and Oliver, M. (1996). *Disability politics: Understanding our past, changing our future.* London and New York: Routledge.

Caudill, W. (1958). *The psychiatric hospital as a small society.* Cambridge, MA: Harvard University Press.

Charlton, J. I. (1998). *Nothing about us without us: Disability oppression and empowerment.* Berkeley: University of California Press.

Coles, G. (2003). *Reading the naked truth: Literacy, legislation, and lies.* Portsmouth, NH: Heinemann.

Conrad, P. (1976). *Identifying hyperactive children: The medicalization of deviant behavior.* Lexington, MA: Lexington Books.

Conrad, P., and Schneider, J. W. (1992). *Deviance and medicalization: From badness to sickness.* Philadelphia: Temple University Press.

Corker, M., and Shakespeare, T. (Eds.). (2002). *Disability/postmodernity: Embodying disability theory.* New York: Continuum.

Davis, F. (1963). *Passage through crisis: Polio victims and their families.* New York: The Bobbs-M errill Company, Inc.

Davis, L. J. (Ed.). (1997). *The Disability Studies reader.* New York and London: Routledge.

Davis, L. J. (2002). *Bending over backwards: Disability, dismodernism & other difficult positions* [Cultural Front]. New York: NYU Press.

Deutsch, H., and Nussbaum, F. (Eds.). (2000). *"Defects": Engendering the modern body* [Corporealities: Discourses of Disability]. Ann Arbor: University of Michigan Press.

Dicker, S. (1990). *Stepping stones: Successful advocacy for children.* New York: Foundation for Child Development.

Douglas, J. D. (Ed.). (1972). *Research on deviance.* New York: Random House.

Dulberger, J. A. (1996). *"Mother donit for the best": Correspondence of a nineteenth-century orphan asylum.* Syracuse, NY: Syracuse University Press.

Dwyer, E. (1987). *Homes for the mad: Life inside two nineteenth-century asylums.* New Brunswick, NJ: Rutgers University Press.

Dybwad, G. (1964). *Challenges in mental retardation.* New York and London: Columbia University Press.

Edgerton, R. B. (1993). *The cloak of competence, revised and updated.* Berkeley: University of California Press.

Eiesland, N. L. (1994). *The disabled God: Toward a liberatory theology of disability.* Nashville: Abingdon Press.

Ellis, C. (1995). *Final negotiations: A story of love, loss, and chronic illness* [Health, Society, and Policy Series]. Philadelphia: Temple University Press.

Evans, R. W. (2004). *The social studies wars: What should we teach the children?* New York: Teachers College Press.

Falk, G. (2001). *Stigma: How we treat outsiders.* Amherst, NY: Prometheus Books.

Farber, B. (1968). *Mental retardation: Its social context and social consequences.* New York: Houghton Miffin Company.

Ferguson, P. M., and Olson, D. (Eds.). (1989, April). *Supported community life: Connecting policy to practice in disability research* [Reports from the Consortium on Youth and Disability Policy]. Eugene, OR: Specialized Training Program, University of Oregon.

Ferri, B. A., and Connor, D. J. (2006). *Reading resistance: Discourses of exclusion in desegregation and inclusion debates* [Disability Studies in Education Vol. 1]. New York: Peter Lang Publishing Group.

Fine, M., and Asch, A. (1988). *Women with disabilities: Essays in psychology, culture, and politics* [Health, Society, and Policy Series]. Philadelphia: Temple University Press.

Finke, B. (2003). *Long time, no see.* Urbana and Chicago: University of Illinois Press.

Fleischer, D. J., and Zames, F. (2001). *The disability rights movement: From charity to confrontation.* Philadelphia: Temple University Press.

Frank, G. (2000). *Venus on wheels: Two decades of dialogue on disability, biography, and being female in America.* Berkeley: University of California Press.

Freeberg, E. (2001). *The education of Laura Bridgman: First deaf and blind person to learn language.* Cambridge, MA and London: Harvard University Press.

Gallagher, D. J., Heshusius, L., Iano, R. P., and Skrtic, T. M. (2004). *Challenging orthodoxy in special education: Dissenting voices.* Denver: Love Publishing Company.

Gaventa, W. C., and Coulter, D. L. (Eds.). (2001). *The theological voice of Wolf Wolfensberger.* Binghamton: The Haworth Pastoral Press, Inc.

Gitlin, T. (1995). *The twilight of common dreams: Why America is wracked by culture wars.* New York: Henry Holt and Company.

Goode, D. (1994). *A world without words: The social construction of children born deaf and blind* [Health, Society, and Policy Series]. Philadelphia: Temple University Press.

Goffman, E. (1961). *Asylums: Essays on the social situation of mental patients and other inmates.* Garden City, NY: Anchor Books.

Goffman, E. (1963). *Stigma: Notes on the management of spoiled identity.* New York: Touchstone.

Groce, N. (1986, May). *"The town fool": An oral history of a mentally retarded individual in small town society* [Wenner-Gren Foundation Working Papers in Anthropology]. New York: Wenner-Gren Foundation.

Groce, N. (1985). *Everyone here spoke sign language: Hereditary deafness on Martha's Vineyard.* Cambridge, MA: Harvard University Press.

Handler, L. (1998). *Twitch and shout: A Touretter's tale.* New York: Plume.

Henry, J. (1973). *Pathways to madness.* New York: Vintage Books.

Herr, S. S., Gostin, L. O., & Koh, H. H. (Eds.). (2003). *The human rights of persons with intellectual disabilities: Different but equal.* Oxford and New York: Oxford University Press.

Higgins, P. C. (1980). *Outsiders in a hearing world: A sociology of deafness* (Sociological Observations). Beverly Hills, CA: Sage Publications.

Ingstad, B., and Whyte, S. R. (Eds.). (1995). *Disability and culture.* Berkeley: University of California Press.

Jacobs, J. (1971). *Adolescent suicide* [Wiley Series on Psychological Disorders]. New York: Wiley-Interscience.

Jenkins, R. (Ed.). (1998). *Questions of competence: Culture, classification and intellectual disability.* Cambridge, UK: Cambridge University Press.

Jodelet, D. (1991). *Madness and social representations: Living with the mad in one French community* [Medicine and Society Vol. 5]. Berkeley: University of California Press.

Johnson, M. (2003). *Make them go away: Clint Eastwood, Christopher Reeve & the case against disability rights.* Louisville, KY: The Advocado Press.

Johnstone, D. (1998). *An introduction to Disability Studies.* London: David Fulton Publishers.

Judge David L. Bazelon Center for Mental Health Law. (2002). *Civil rights and human dignity: Three decades of leadership in advocacy for people with mental disabilities.* Washington, DC: Author.

Karp, D. A. (1996). *Speaking of sadness: Depression, disconnection, and the meanings of illness.* Oxford and New York: Oxford University Press.

Kluth, P., Straut, D. M., and Biklen, D. (Eds.). (2003). *Access to academics for all students: Critical approaches to inclusive curriculum, instruction, and policy.* Mahwah, NJ: Lawrence Erlbaum Associates.

Krieger, L.H. (2003). *Backlash against the ADA: Reinterpreting disability rights* [Corporealities: Discourses of Disability]. Ann Arbor, MI: University of Michigan Press.

Lane, H. (1999). *The mask of benevolence: Disabling the Deaf community* (2nd ed.). San Diego: Dawn Sign Press.

Lantzy, M. L. (1992). *Individuals with Disabilities Education Act: An annotated guide to its literature and resources, 1980-1991.* Littleton, CO: Fred B. Rothman & Co.

Linneman, R. D. (2001). *Idiots: Stories about mindedness and mental retardation* [Counterpoints: Studies in the Postmodern Theory of Education Vol. 154]. New York: Peter Lang Publishing.

Linton, S. (1998). *Claiming disability: Knowledge and identity* (Cultural Front). New York: New York University Press.

Longmore, P. K. (2003). *Why I burned my book and other essays on disability* (American Subjects). Philadelphia: Temple University Press.

Longmore, P. K., and Umansky, L. (Eds.). (2001). *The new disability history: American perspectives* [The History of Disability]. New York: New York University Press.

Lyman, K. A. (1993). *Day in, day out with Alzheimer's: Stress in caregiving relationships* [Health, Society, and Policy Series]. Philadelphia: Temple University Press.

Makas, E., and Schlesinger, L. (Eds.). (1996). *End results and starting points: Expanding the field of Disability Studies.* Portland, ME: The Society for Disability Studies & The Edmund S. Muskie Institute of Public Affairs.

Minow, M. (1990). *Making all the difference: Inclusion, exclusion, and American law.* Ithaca, NY: Cornell University Press.

Mitchell, D. T., and Snyder, S. L. (Eds.). (1997). *The body and physical difference: Discourses of disability* [The Body, In Theory: Histories of Cultural Materialism]. Ann Arbor: University of Michigan Press.

Murphy, R. F. (1987). *The body silent: An anthropologist embarks on the most challenging journey of his life: Into the world of the disabled.* London and New York: W.W. Norton.

Murphy, S. T., and Rogan, P. M. (1995). *Closing the shop: Conversion from sheltered to integrated work.* Baltimore: Paul H. Brookes Publis hing Co.

Nagler, M. (Ed.). *Perspectives on disability: Text and readings on disability.* Palo Alto, CA: Health Markets Research.

Nyiszli, M. (1960). *Auschwitz: A doctor's eyewitness account.* New York: Arcade Publishing.

O'Brien, R. (2001). *Crippled justice: The history of modern disability policy in the workplace.* Chicago: University of Chicago Press.

Olson, L. K. (2003). *The not-so-golden years: Caregiving, the frail eldery, and the long-term care establishment.* Lanham, MD: Rowman & Littlefield Publishers, Inc.

Pelka, F. (1997). *The ABC-CLIO companion to the disability rights movement.* Santa Barbara, CA: ABC-CLIO.

Perlin, M. L., Kanter, A., Treuthart, M. P., Szeli, E., and Gledhill, K. (Eds.). (2006). *International human rights and comparative mental disability law: Cases and materials.* Durham, NC: Carolina Academic Press.

Pernick, M. S. (1996). *The black stork: Eugenics and the death of "defective" babies in American medicine and motion pictures since 1915.* Oxford and New York: Oxford University Press, Inc.

Pointon, A., and Davies, C. (Eds.). (1997). *Framed: Interrogating disability in the media.* London: British Film Institute.

Priestley, M. (2003). *Disability: A life course approach.* Cambridge, UK: Polity.

Radical Teacher, No. 47: Disability studies (Feature issue). (1995, Fall). Somerville, MA: Boston Women's Teachers' Group, Inc.

Ritzer, G. (1998). *The McDonaldization thesis: Explorations and extensions.* Thousand Oaks, CA: Sage Publications.

Robillard, A. B. (1999). *Meaning of a disability: The lived experience of paralysis.* Philadelphia: Temple University Press.

Rogers, L. J., and Swadener, B. B. (Eds.). (2001). *Semiotics & Dis/ability: Interrogating categories of difference.* Albany: State University of New York press.

Roosens, E. (1979). *Mental patients in town life: Geel—Europe's first therapeutic community* [Sage Library of Social Research Vol. 90]. Beverly Hills: Sage Publications.

osen, G. (1968). *Madness in society: Chapters in the historical sociology of mental illness.* New York: Harper Torchbooks.

Rosenthal, E., Kanter, A. *et al.* (2003, September 9). *Foreign policy and disability: Legislative strategies and civil rights protections to ensure inclusion of people with disabilities.* Washington, DC: National Council on Disability.

Roth, J. A., and Eddy, E. M. (1967). *Rehabilitation for the unwanted.* New York: Atherton Press.

Rothman, D. J., and Rothman, S. M. (1984). *The Willowbrook wars: A decade of struggle for social justice.* New York: Harper & Row, Publishers.

Russell, M. (1998). *Beyond ramps: Disability at the end of the social contract.* Monroe, ME: Common Courage Press.

Ryan, D. F., and Schuchman, J. S. (Eds.). (2002). *Deaf people in Hitler's Europe.* Washington, DC: Gallaudet University Press in association with the United States Holocaust Memorial Museum.

Ryan, W. (1976). *Blaming the victim* (Rev. ed.). New York: Vintage.

Sacks, O. (1990). *Seeing voices: A journey into the world of the Deaf.* New York: Harper Perennial.

Safford, P. L., and Safford, E. J. (1996). *A history of childhood & disability.* New York: Teachers College Press.

Sarason, S. B. (1996). *Revisiting "The culture of the school and the problem of change"* [The Series on School Reform]. New York: Teachers College Press.

Sarason, S. B., and Doris, J. (1979). *Educational handicap, public policy, and social history: A broadened perspective on mental retardation.* New York: Free Press.

Scheerenberger, R. C. (1983). *A history of mental retardation.* Baltimore: Paul H. Brookes Publishing Co.

Scheerenberger, R. C. (1987). *A history of mental retardation: A quarter century of promise.* Baltimore: Paul H. Brookes Publishing Co.

Scheff, T. J. (1999). *Being mentally ill: A sociological theory* (3rd ed.). Hawthorne, NY: Aldine de Gruyter.

Scheff, T. J. (Ed.). (1975). *Labeling madness.* Englewood Cliffs, NJ: Prentice-Hall, Inc.

Schein, J. D. (1989). *At home among strangers: Exploring the Deaf community in the United States.* Washington, DC: Gallaudet University Press.

Schlesinger, L., and Taub, D. E. (Eds.). (1998). *Syllabi and instructional materials for teaching sociology and Disability Studies.* Washington, DC: American Sociological Association.

Schlesinger, L., and Taub, D. E. (Eds.). (2004). *Instructional materials for teaching sociology & Disability Studies* (2nd ed.). Washington, DC: American Sociological Association.

Schnorr, R., Ford, A., Davern, L., Park-Lee, Seunghee, & Meyer, L. (1989). *The Syracuse curriculum revision manual: A group process for developing a community-referenced curriculum guide.* Baltimore: Paul H. Brookes Publishing Co.

Scott, R.A. (1969). *The making of blind men: A study of adult socialization.* New York: Russell Sage Foundation.

Scull, A. (1984). *Decarceration: Community treatment and the deviant – A radical view* (2nd ed.). New Brunswick, NJ: Rutgers University Press.

Shakespeare, T. (Ed.). (1998). *The disability reader: Social science perspectives.* London and New York: Cassell.

Shuttleworth, G. E., and Potts, W. A. (1916). *Mentally deficient children: Their treatment and training* (4th ed.). Philadelphia: P. Blakison's Son & Co.

Silverstein, R. (2000, August). *Emerging disability policy framework: A guidepost for analyzing public policy.* Iowa Law Review, 85, 1691-2000.

Skrtic, T. M. (1991). *Behind special education: A critical analysis of professional culture and school organization.* Denver: Love Publishing Company.

Skrtic, T. M. (Ed.). (1995). *Disability & democracy: Reconstructing (special) education for postmodernity* [Special Education Series]. New York: Teachers College Press.

Smith, R. C. (1996). *A case about Amy* [Health, Society, and Policy]. Philadelphia: Temple University Press.

Smoller, E. S. (1997). *"I can't remember": Family stories of Alzheimer's disease.* Philadelphia: Temple University Press.

Snyder, S. L., Brueggemann, B. J., and Garland-Thomson, R. (Eds.). (2002). *Disability studies: Enabling the humanities.* New York: The Modern Language Association of America.

Spradley, T. S., and Spradley, J. P. (1978). *Deaf like me.* New York: Random House.

Stiker, H. (1997). *A history of disability* [Corporealities: Discourses of Disability]. Ann Arbor: University of Michigan Press.

Stroman, D. F. (2003). *The disability rights movement: From deinstitutionalization to self-determination.* Lanham, MD: University Press of America, Inc.

Szasz, T. (Ed.). (1973). *The age of madness: The history of involuntary mental hospitalization presented in selected texts.* Garden City, NY: Anchor Books.

Titchkosky, T. (2003). *Disability, self, and society.* Toronto: University of Toronto Press.

Tredgold, R. F., and Soddy, K. (1963). *Textbook of mental deficiency (subnormality)* (10th ed.). Baltimore: The Williams and Wilkins Co.

Trent, J. W. (1994). *Inventing the feeble mind: A history of mental retardation in the United States* [Medicine in Society]. Berkeley: University of California Press.

Van Cleve, J. V., and Crouch, B. A. (1989). *A place of their own: Creating the Deaf community in America.* Washington, DC: Gallaudet University Press.

Walker, P. M., and Rogan, P. (2007). *Make the day matter! Promoting typical lifestyles for adults with significant disabilities.* Baltimore: Paul H. Brookes Publishing Co.

Wendell, S. (1996). *The rejected body: Feminist philosophical reflections on disability.* London and New York: Routledge.

Williams, P., and Shoultz, B. (1986). *We can speak for ourselves: Self-advocacy by mentally handicapped people.* Bloomington, IN: Indiana University Press.

Wilson, J. C., and Lewiecki-Wilson, C. (2001). *Embodied rhetorics: Disability in language and culture.* Carbondale, IL: Southern Illinois University Press.

Wolfensberger, W. (1972). *The principle of normalization in human services.* Toronto: National Institute on Mental Retardation.

Wolfensberger, W. (1998). *A brief introduction to social role valorization: A high-order concept for addressing the plight of societally devalued people, and for structuring human services* (3rd ed.). Syracuse, NY: The Training Institute for Human Service Planning, Leadership and Change Agentry, Syracuse University.

Wolfensberger, W. (2003). *The future of children with significant impairments: What parents fear and want, and what they and others may be able to do about it.* Syracuse, NY: The Training Institute for Human Service Planning, Leadership and Change Agentry, Syracuse University.

Index